Creating Meaning in Funerals

Creating Meaning in Funerals is a book about the ways in which bereaved families and communities create meaningful ceremonies against a backdrop of what is culturally appropriate, even when their choices might make little economic sense to those outside the culture. The culmination of these customs and practices, this book maintains, is how bereaved individuals, families, and communities are drawn into significant meaning making in early bereavement. Readers will be repeatedly challenged to suspend their own biases, observe the customs and beliefs of others thoughtfully, and provide counseling support and encouragement to bereaved individuals for whom funerals were or were not effective means of coping with their loss.

Discussion questions at the end of each chapter make the book useful for educational settings such as funeral service classroom instruction, thanatology classes, and grief counseling courses. Each chapter is also accompanied by its own reference list to make chapters more useful individually.

William G. Hoy has spent more than 40 years caring for the dying and bereaved and was Clinical Professor of Medical Humanities at Baylor University in Waco, Texas, from 2012 until 2024.

"Not only is *Creating Meaning in Funerals* a great title for a book, it is a theme demonstrated in each chapter. Hoy has written a significant contribution to the field of thanatology and a solid rebuttal of the arguments of funeral critics. Repeatedly, due to the scope of the lit review, as I read —and underlined—I wrote, 'I didn't know that!' I found this a valuable read and will soon re-read it. As they say in Texas, 'This is a good steer!'"

Harold Ivan Smith, *DMin, FT, author of* Borrowed Narratives: Using Biographical and Historical Grief Narratives With the Bereaving

"Dr. Hoy brings a valuable resource to thanatology researchers, practitioners, and educators. Using his signature narrative style, he dives into the value of ceremony and the ways in which bereavement is socially constructed using beautiful, real-life examples. His use of the five anchors from his compass model of grief is superb and links connection to cultural heritage. This book is a must have for everyone working in end-of-life care."

Becky Lomaka, *MA, CT, Director of Grief Support and Education, O'Connor Mortuary, California, USA*

"In this essential book, Bill Hoy draws on his extensive research and clinical practice to offer us insight into the many ways people find meaning and direction through the ceremonial anchors of funeral rituals. Along the way we learn about different approaches to funerals around the world. The illustrative stories help us understand the ways ceremonies can help us all as we move through grief after a significant death. It is a book everyone should read."

Janet E. McCord, *PhD, FT, Professor of Thanatology, Edgewood College, Wisconsin, USA*

Creating Meaning in Funerals

How Families and Communities Make Sense of Death

William G. Hoy

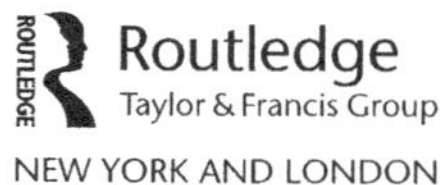

NEW YORK AND LONDON

Designed cover image: Marharyta Fatieieva © Getty Images

First published 2025
by Routledge
605 Third Avenue, New York, NY 10158

and by Routledge
4 Park Square, Milton Park, Abingdon, Oxon OX14 4RN

Routledge is an imprint of the Taylor & Francis Group, an informa business

ISBN: 978-1-032-39837-2 (hbk)
ISBN: 978-1-032-39832-7 (pbk)
ISBN: 978-1-003-35301-0 (ebk)

DOI: 10.4324/9781003353010

Typeset in Optima
by Taylor & Francis Books

Contents

About the Author

With more than 40 years in caring for the dying and bereaved through congregation, hospice, and bereavement center, William G. Hoy was clinical professor of medical humanities at Baylor University from 2012 to 2024. He was the recipient of the Association for Death Education's Academic Educator of the Year award in 2021. In his retirement, he sees a few patients and seeks to help enhance the skills of colleagues in this work through his frequent presentations and writing.

Although primarily a bedside clinician, Dr. Hoy has authored more than 200 articles and book chapters; this is his seventh book. His books in print include *Do Funerals Matter? The Purposes and Practices of Death Rituals in Global Perspective* (Routledge, 2013) and *Bereavement Groups and the Role of Social Support: Integrating Theory, Research, and Practice* (Routledge, 2016).

He is widely regarded as an authority on the role of social support in death, dying, and grief. His work has included extensive and respectful ethnographic perspectives on the social support afforded to African American families and communities through traditional "homegoing" ceremonies and, for many years, has been interested in the interplay of poverty and funeral choice among low-resource people groups. He has done extensive fieldwork on the Nyakach Plateau of rural western Kenya.

Dr. Hoy is active in the Association for Death Education and Counseling on whose board he served from 2012 to 2020 including six years as an officer. He holds the Fellow in Thanatology (F.T.), the highest level of board certification in thanatology, and he serves on the advisory board and as a frequent author and program contributor for the Tragedy Assistance Program for Survivors (T.A.P.S.) in Washington, D.C. In his retirement, he is a frequent contributor to the Hospice Foundation of America's *Journeys* monthly newsletter for bereaved individuals.

Foreword

Louis A. Gamino, Ph.D., A.B.P.P., F.T.

Every human being dies. Nothing in our contemporary world changes this immutable fact, regardless of how sophisticated we may view ourselves and our cultures. That reality of inevitable death poses ever-present challenges of what to do with the deceased person's body and how to cope with the loss of that person's physical presence in our lives. In this volume, Dr. Hoy addresses the perennial questions and issues that arise pertaining to funerals, memorializations, and life after death for survivors of the deceased. Because we cannot escape death, the contents of a book like this one never go out of style.

Despite advances in the death awareness movement, as well as a burgeoning scholarly literature on dying and grief, it sometimes appears that postmodern society has persisted in its preference to ignore, forestall, or just plain deny the reality of human mortality. This denial may actually be facilitated by various options for disposition of the body now available to mourners. Beyond time-honored traditions like casketing followed by earth burial or ceremonial cremation then dispersion in a sacred river, contemporary mourners embrace a multitude of choices. Some may opt for immediate cremation but defer permanent disposition to a later time and place (if ever); meanwhile the loved one's cremains stay on a closet shelf out of sight to avoid the discomfort of thinking about the loss. Alternately, a variety of jewelry or ornamental pieces may contain cremains to acknowledge or celebrate the ongoing presence of loved ones who can be seen and felt right here now. Environmentally influenced choices like composting the deceased's body to grow a tree may support the idea that the deceased loved one is not really gone but lives on in a tangibly evident way. The latest twist comes from the world of artificial intelligence (A.I.) where software engineers create digital avatars of the deceased loved one. These virtual impersonations are designed to interact in real time with survivors, simulating the deceased person's voice and movements, therefore making it possible to "maintain your bond forever." Embedded in all these practices seems to be the unspoken illusion, "If my loved one never really died, maybe I won't have to die either."

Sometimes denial exhibits itself in the choice not to hold any sort of service acknowledging a loved one's death. I recall the neighbor who saw me in the yard one day and took that occasion to quietly tell me his wife had died months before, as if to explain why she had not been seen recently—no obituary, no funeral, no public acknowledgment of her death, almost as if she had never lived. I was stunned by his news. Rationalizations abound for such decisions. Mourners may cite the fact that the deceased person "didn't want any service," completely discounting the obvious sociological fact that funerals are needed for the living to say goodbye, express their grief, and receive much needed support and reassurance from the community of the living. Lack of specific religious beliefs or an inability to afford a funeral can also be heard as rationales for skipping services altogether. Often underlying such choices is not only denial of death but also a convenient avoidance of grief, as if by closing one's eyes and heart to the death, it is possible to "take a pass" on experiencing any emotional pain or distress.

Irvin Yalom (1980) thoughtfully reminded us, "The physicality of death destroys us but the idea of death saves us" (p. 40). Only by living our lives with full awareness that we are finite creatures, allotted limited time on planet Earth, can we truly live authentically and vibrantly, fully appreciating the gift of our existence. Individuals who are existentially aware in this manner recognize death for what it is, prepare for it, deal with it when it happens, and use the experience to enhance their understanding of life and inform the choices they make. Readers of this volume will learn innumerable ways to help grieving people face inevitable death with grace and courage, in the process promoting their psychological and emotional adaptation to loss.

With wisdom and eloquence reflecting decades of experience in end-of-life work, Dr. Hoy systematically and persuasively argues how carefully crafted funerals and memorializations honor the deceased person in a meaningful manner that jump-starts the all-important psychological task of integrating the reality of that loss into the rest of the mourner's life. Incorporating his previous work on the five anchors of funeral rituals (Chapter 1) as well as his highly accessible compass model of grief (Chapter 2), Hoy shows readers how to design meaningful funerals and memorial services that lay a foundation for subsequent healthy adaptation. Consistent with many psychotherapy approaches based on reversing unhealthy avoidance, Hoy encourages death professionals to gently guide bereft persons through the headwinds of early grief as they confront the necessary tasks of dealing with the deceased person's body and planning services, all the while maintaining fidelity to the core values that inform their lives. With Hoy's approach, denial and avoidance are not in charge.

One of the main benefits death professionals will realize from reading this book is to learn how best to serve surviving families and loved ones at a critical point in time when survivors' own executive processes may be compromised by the emotional impact of the death. A helpful section on clinical implications concludes each chapter in the book, along with the many creative ideas shared throughout the manuscript. Taken together, these materials form a very useful primer for professional helpers who need knowledge of what is possible by way of funerals and memorializations in order to best assist grieving families and loved ones in making meaningful choices.

This book is not just for professionals working in funeral homes or clergy who interact with families *at the time of death*, although they certainly can fully utilize its content during arrangement planning conferences and interactions with grieving families. Sometimes health-care professionals, such as those working in clinics, hospitals, hospices, palliative care units, or nursing care facilities, have the opportunity to inform or empower families grappling with a loved one's *impending death* and wondering how they will manage it. Planning and preparing how to cope is a fundamental tenet of psychological resilience. Finally, mental health professionals frequently encounter cases of individuals struggling *after the death* of a treasured loved one, often due to problems with prolonged grief disorder. In some instances, family conflicts or lack of opportunity to participate in funeral decisions have left certain grievers without a chance to say goodbye on their own terms or genuinely perform leave-taking in a suitable manner. Yet, it is never too late. The wonderful ideas contained in this book may still be applied afterward, in personally meaningful rituals that discharge the basic human obligations to bury the dead but never forget.

How Dr. Hoy worked with the grieving mother described at the end of Chapter 6 by reading aloud in the consultation room the eulogy she had written for her deceased son—but never given the opportunity to deliver because there were no services—is a fine example of a clinically sensitive, well-timed, innovative application of good funeral practices transposed to a mental health setting. In my experience, this kind of intervention is rarely discussed in graduate curricula or clinical training, yet can achieve so much good when treating complicated grief. Tools of this type and much more await the reader open to learning the principles and methods taught in Dr. Hoy's book.

Pondering the possibilities for meaning inherent in each and every funeral or memorialization brings to mind a story shared by retired funeral director Rick Bissler, who for decades owned and operated Bissler and Sons Funeral Home in Kent, Ohio. When a beloved local repairman died, his family came to the planning conference having already decided on cremation. Rick had to admit that nowhere in his many catalogs of urns was a receptable that fittingly honored the deceased man and how he had spent his life. Instead, with the family's permission, Rick approached the man's HVAC coworkers and suggested they fabricate a "toolbox" urn in which to place his cremains. Besides engraving the deceased man's name and birth/death dates on the front of the steel box, each of his fellow shopworkers engraved their name on the back as a tribute to their trusted colleague. The family did likewise. At the deceased man's memorial service, an elegantly simple table covered with a white linen cloth featuring his tool belt, the toolbox urn, and a single vase of flowers said it all. This kind of creativity not only made for a superbly meaningful memorial service but also afforded the mourners a sorely needed kinesthetic outlet for expressing their grief and honoring the deceased man's legacy in a fashion they would always remember. Would that every final service be that respectful, consoling, and memorable.

Reference

Yalom, I.D. (1980). *Existential psychotherapy*. New York: Basic.

Preface

William G. Hoy https://orcid.org/0000-0001-6118-1261

I was born into a family in grief. In addition to three living children, my mother had suffered two miscarriages before my birth. Having been born during the early Roaring 20s, my parents lived out their childhood in the throes of the Great Depression, and my mother's father died when she was only 11. At my birth, it had been barely a year since our family had bid farewell to my beloved paternal grandmother who died of cancer in the days when there were virtually no treatment options; I was conceived in grief.

For his own part, my father, a veteran of World War II, had seen his share of buddies killed. But the one that struck him and our family the hardest, undoubtedly, was that of his only brother who died in the war in 1943. Although his body was never recovered, we were reminded of Marshall's death at every patriotic holiday in my childhood because my grandfather, who lived just across the road from us, displayed the flag given to him and my grandmother by the War Department before there was a Veterans Administration.

Loss in our family had not caused the clinical impairment that we would come six decades later to call prolonged grief disorder, but unmistakably, grief colored much of how our family functioned. Only later would I realize it could not have been otherwise. So, one could say, not only did I live my early life adjacent to death, but in a real sense, death and grief are deeply woven into my DNA.

Apparently, my interest in death rituals started early. In the family archives is a badly faded picture from the early 1960s, an unposed photo my father captured of me leaning over and peering intently at a tombstone emblazoned with the surname Hoy in an overgrown graveyard. The rural cemetery in Quebec was the final resting place for several of our family in their new adopted homeland when they immigrated from Scotland in the mid-19th century. Actually, my great-grandfather, a pirate according to family lore, was apparently deported to Canada, but that is a story for another time.

Funerals course through my blood. As a church organist through high school and most of college, I provided music for more funerals than I can count. They were conveniently on school days, allowing me to skip classes, and I was almost always paid a small honorarium, my first experience with getting "two for one." Along the way, I was also training for a life in pastoral ministry.

During the early days of that training, my mentor took me to the National Conference on Preaching being held nearby; Baptist pastors of that generation attended such meetings. In one of the plenary sessions, I heard a well-regarded minister explain with confidence how he did not like having caskets at church for funerals, that he personally preferred cremation, and that when the family insisted on burial, it should, in his wise counsel, be held before the memorial service so the family could "focus on the Lord and not the corpse." Even to my young, inexperienced pastoral mind, his advice seemed oddly out of step with how bereaved individuals experience loss.

With college complete, I served as an associate pastor in one of the oldest congregations of my denomination in the state of California while I attended seminary. There were a lot of funerals. All the while, my conviction intensified that how we memorialize our dead is somehow related to how we grieve. A decade later in my second congregation and well into my first "lead pastor" role, I was an on-call pastor for a couple of local funeral directors, so funerals became my constant companion as I walked with several dozen families through that experience every year.

I loved that ministry, and most people around me seemed to think I was good at it, though honestly, I was way out of my professional depth. With its 90 semester hours of work beyond the baccalaureate degree, the master of divinity degree includes more than 4,000 hours of classroom study plus uncountable hours of reading and writing. I have discovered I am not alone in reporting that in that entire formal education, we had one 60-minute lecture about grief and funerals. Fortunately, Johnny Wilson, my favorite Old Testament professor and a brilliant pastor-scholar, led an optional seminar for a few of us in the pastoral use of the Psalms, and I got lots of tips from him.

So it is little surprise I would return to school to focus on grief and loss and, within a short time, would leave congregational leadership to concentrate on care of the dying and bereaved, first as a hospice chaplain and eventually for a total of 17 years at the helm of the bereavement program for Pathways Volunteer Hospice in the multicultural milieu of Long Beach, California. In those days, our public school district was populated by children whose families spoke more than 100 languages at home. I learned to care for the dying and bereaved in a place where there was intense diversity.

Soon, I realized that despite the unique customs of every major religion and ethnic group represented in our community, there were some universals that bound humans together in the face of death, regardless of the language we spoke, the religious beliefs that gave us meaning, and the cultural customs we observed. Discovering what those anchors were set me on a parallel track of research, even during my busy clinical practice. Those discoveries were chronicled in a book many years later, *Do Funerals Matter? The Purposes and Practices of Death Rituals in Global Perspective* (Routledge, 2013).

Gratefully, that volume has enjoyed a great reception from reviewers, scholars, fellow clinicians, and teachers alike with many utilizing the text in their own survey courses on death and dying. Using funerals as the comparison point has proven to be a helpful way to teach cultural awareness to my own pre-health students at Baylor University over the last several years. But even though funeral customs change at a glacially slow pace, the book needed to be updated or expanded. In my conversations with Anna Moore, my tireless acquisitions editor at Routledge, it became clear that although we *could* produce a second edition, the contents of this volume really are a whole new book. Thus, *Creating Meaning in Funerals* was born.

This volume therefore further expands my thinking from the earlier volume and updates it with the challenges we face socially and clinically in the third decade of the 21st century. When the first book was published, we knew nothing about the COVID-19 pandemic that swept across the globe changing lives and challenging funeral customs. And on economic fronts, we know more—and are more conscious—about the great gap between people who live in high-resource and low-resource communities. These also have a dramatic impact on funerals but not in the ways politicians and development experts have often assumed.

For the last dozen years, my professional role has been as a clinical professor in the Medical Humanities Program at Baylor University, where I had the rare privilege of helping the next generation of young physicians and other health-care professionals learn about the intersection of loss with health. Now I have retired from that post to focus the last years of my career once again on caring for the bereaved and in enhancing the skills of my caregiving colleagues in counseling the bereaved.

So this volume updates what I have learned and continue to discover from bereaved individuals about the role of ceremonies in "acting out" their grief. The book updates the anchors of memorial ceremonies described in the 2013 volume, connecting these to the grief process and the vital role of social support. Here, readers will also find descriptions of grief and how funerals are utilized when children die, as well as how funerals are related to the complicators of grief such as traumatic accidents, substance overdoses, suicides, and homicides.

The COVID-19 pandemic changed health and economic well-being around the globe, and those challenges were felt most acutely among bereaved individuals and communities who were often restricted from their most helpful rituals employed in facing early grief. Although this volume expands the earlier volume's descriptions of religious and cultural traditions in memorial ceremonies, it focuses especially on how African Americans have employed funerals in bereavement despite deep economic challenges and the health disparities laid bare by the pandemic.

Uses of Cases and Names

Clinicians and researchers alike find great challenge in making decisions about when and under what circumstances to use the names and stories of real people, recognizing that the narratives represented in cases make the content come alive. However, my students and I have declared in our myriad applications to Baylor's Institutional Review Board that the names and identifying information of research participants would never be disclosed in our published reports, and I honor those promises here. The professionals I have interviewed are identified only by their specialty and, when necessary, the vocational characteristics that qualify them to offer the perspectives they do.

I have been equally cautious with the stories of bereaved people, changing identities and specific information about causes and circumstances of death, family dynamics, and other complex features of the cases. Obviously, that means some of the more sensational details have been diluted, but the educational value of those added details do not justify the possible violation of professional confidence. Only when names are widely known in the media or in previously published work (such as with celebrity funerals), or in cases where I am describing funerals in my own family, where I report details without fear of breaking a confidence, have I taken the liberty to name individuals and describe in unaltered detail the ceremonies that honor the lives of real people.

In Gratitude

Books might bear the sole author's name, but they are almost never truly the product of one person. Countless individuals have told me their stories—hundreds of times in clinical conversations, frequently in the moments following a seminar, and sometimes in research interviews. These people include many bereaved individuals who, through both group settings and individual conversations, answered my clinical questions like, "Tell me about the funeral" and "What worked for you, what did not work for you?" and "What do you most remember about the words that were spoken or the songs that were sung or the people who were there?" and "What would you change about the memorial ceremony if you could?" I have always found these to be fruitful ways to get inside a person's grief and, more often than anyone wants to admit, are often the keys to discovering what has gone awry with the person's experience with bereavement to set up what we call in our guild *prolonged grief disorder*.

Therefore, here I express my deepest gratitude to these patients as well as the dozens of professionals—clergy, funeral directors, social workers, and bereavement counselors—who have so unselfishly and transparently offered their stories and experiences. Although in honoring the guarantees my students and I made to the Institutional Review Board to not identify research participants, my eternal gratitude is due to these individuals who so willingly told their stories. We often promised a 20-minute interview that lasted two hours, I believe in part because people long to be heard. Nevertheless, this volume would be just a shadow of itself if not for the willingness and transparency with which these individuals have offered their lives and perspectives.

Then, of course, there are my colleagues at Baylor during these years—Lauren Barron, Jason Whitt, Bill Nielson, Helen Harris, Sparky Matthews, Lisa Baker, Jim Marcum, David Stamile, James Ellor, and Sheila Smith. In countless conversations and the collegiality that is known among clinicians and scholars who make their lives in the academy, these people have influenced all my work in ways that I could not fully catalog even if I tried. To them, I owe an undying sense of gratitude.

Perhaps among my professional colleagues, two groups of people rise to the surface most notably who have influenced my life and my work—my friends in funeral service and my colleagues in the Association for Death Education and Counseling (A.D.E.C.). Among the former group are people like Randy Stricklin, Neil O'Connor, Becky Lomaka, Rick Bissler, Chad Snyder, Hatch Bailey, and two generations of the McAfee family—Tommy, John, and Jay. What I understand about funeral customs and options has had a fine point put on it by these consummate professionals who have tirelessly cared for their communities, often at great personal risk and sacrifice, especially during times like the global pandemic explored in Chapter 7.

Like many of my colleagues in the death and grief space, for nearly 35 years, I have called A.D.E.C. my professional home. Louis Gamino, Janet McCord, Ken Doka, Ben Wolfe, Bob Neimeyer, Brenda Atkinson, Galen Goben, Rebecca Morse, Harold Ivan Smith, and Fay Green are not just professional colleagues; they are dear friends whose work has been instrumental in my own thinking and writing through the decades. Many of these people have read all or parts of this manuscript along with countless other papers and book chapters before they ever saw the light of day. I am beyond grateful for your kindness, your helpfulness, and your friendship, though errors in this book are mine alone.

When I was a young counselor, fresh out of grad school, I knew I needed more in-depth training than my graduate education and supervision had afforded me, especially in the area of caring for the dying and bereaved in an evidence-informed clinical model. In graduate school, I realized how behind we were in that a professor called up Kübler-Ross's five stages as the model for bereavement care even though I already knew during that 1985 class there had been better evidence-based models around for more than a decade. That was my first exposure to the notion that just because an educator "professes" knowledge does not always mean he or she has kept up, especially in a field tangential to his or her own academic training or clinical work.

When writing my senior sociology thesis on the social ramifications of death in American society years earlier, I discovered J. William Worden's newly published work, *Grief Counseling and Grief Therapy: A Handbook for the Mental Health Practitioner*. I was immediately taken by Worden's clinically informed, evidence-based thinking and soon found it practical in my work with grieving people. So when I realized this hero had moved from his Harvard appointment in Boston to Rosemead School of Psychology in Southern California, and he invited me to be part of his supervision group for advanced therapists, I jumped at the chance. Across these decades, Bill has moved in my mind and heart from hero to mentor to colleague to friend, and his influence on my life and work is incalculable. I realize Bill has been my colleague and friend through all the revisions to that volume, culminating in the fifth edition published in 2018 and as we have watched the page count grow from 146 to its present 292, still brief by any standard.

Finally, this book would not have been possible without the tireless devotion of my family. My adult children, Carolyn and Greg, endured far more stops at cemeteries and museums during their childhood and teenage years than any children should expect, but they always did it with grace and patience—or at least that is how I recall those trips now. It has been a joy to watch the two of them flourish into amazing lives. Even as a compassionate physician-scientist in the midst of his training, Greg took time from his work in Paris to visit Père Lachaise and its amazing catacombs and then to discover and send to me an thorough history of the social meanings of the place, Erin-Marie Legacey's *Making Space for the Dead*.

Our daughter, Carolyn, spent the first chapter of her career as a professional writer and now is performing the most vital work of a full-time wife to Matthew and mom to our amazing grandchildren, Sydney and Nick. Carolyn found lots of late nights after the kids were in bed to serve as my editor and tirelessly made hundreds of suggestions to improve my writing that often too much resembles how I talk. This book would not be nearly as good without her endless devotion to that task. Thank you.

Debbie has been my constant companion, wife, and best friend for more than 36 years. She has seen me through more than her share of "those" periods when my writing took precedence over things she would rather us do together. When I signed the contract to write this book, we were caring for Deb's mother in our home during the last years of her life. So our own experience with bereavement has been, in many ways, a laboratory for learning and discovery on what it means to use ceremonies old and new to create meaning in loss, and I am beyond honored to tell the story of Margaret's funeral in Chapter 1.

In Memoriam

In the years since *Do Funerals Matter? The Purposes and Practices of Death Rituals in Global Perspective* was published in 2013, our family has walked through many deaths and the rituals that accompany them. I am so grateful that my extended family has consistently refused to embrace the "simpler is better" motif in funerals that has seemed to dominate our age. In addition to my mother-in-law, Margaret, mentioned earlier, Debbie and I have now buried all four parents with her dad and my mom dying just seven weeks apart in 2016. Then my family was rocked by the surprising—and not—death of my 39-year-old nephew Daniel, right in the middle of the pandemic in July 2020 when he died after more than three decades living with Duchenne muscular dystrophy.

Only 13 months later, his dad and my brother, Don, died at the age of 63, thrusting our family once again into the abyss of bereavement in which funerals play a vital role in helping us to begin creating meaning. Along with my father, Edwin Willis Hoy, who died in 1993 when I was still quite green, yet in the first decade of my own career, all of these people—William (Bill) E. Coffey, Lillie Mae Hoy, Daniel Ray Hoy, Donald Ray Hoy, and Margaret Jean Coffey—have helped make this volume what it is, and I honor them for that deep contribution. Most of all, however, these people contributed immeasurably to my life and the lives of countless others, not just in their deaths but, most important, in the way they lived their lives. I dedicate this book to these wonderful forebears who have, by their lives and deaths, shown us how life is done well.

Introduction

Although it is not the first funeral ever recorded in writing, the Hebrew Bible's first book, B'reshith (Genesis in the Christian Old Testament), ends with a stirring account of the dying declarations and blessings on his sons by the patriarch Jacob. Before his death, Jacob asked his sons to make sure that his body was not interred in the land of Egypt but rather that his remains be returned to Canaan, the "land of promise" (Genesis 49:29–32). Then the narrator turns to a lengthy description of the burial ceremonies held for this patriarch who is honored in Judaism, Christianity, and Islam.

Much of the final chapter of Genesis is devoted to describing these observances. If there are ritual prayers offered, music sung, or a eulogy delivered during the funeral ceremonies themselves, the biblical text makes no mention of them. Rather, the funeral follows a simply prescribed ritual of preparation of the body, gathering of extended family and presumably close friends, and a long deliberate procession through the wilderness. The body's preparation, readers are told, needed 40 days, and either following that or concurrently with that preparation, the people mourned 70 days (Genesis 50:3). The procession to Caanan likely required an additional two weeks, including a lengthy stop along the way, as the people reached Atad, just inside the borders of the Promised Land: "They lamented there with a very great and grievous lamentation, and he made a mourning for his father seven days" (Genesis 50:10 ESV). This is the first recorded occurrence of the Hebrew people "sitting shiva," a custom observed among traditional Jews in the 21st century (Popovsky, 2007).

Like many records from antiquity, funerals in Hebrew history are often described in great detail with an eye to their most important characteristics. Even a casual observer notes that the ceremonies surrounding death are important in the Jacob narrative. The textual record of the deathbed blessing of his children and the funeral proceedings occupy approximately one-fifth of the entire biography of Jacob's life as told in the scriptures shared by Jews and Christians. Because ancient people went to such effort to describe their funerals and because contemporary people seem to place so much emphasis on how lives are remembered

DOI: 10.4324/9781003353010-1

after a death, it seems appropriate to explore the mechanism whereby families and communities utilize these death ceremonies to begin making meaning of their losses.

Creating Meaning in Funerals takes as its primary goal increasing this understanding of a host of professional and volunteer caregivers so that bereaved individuals are cared for more effectively. This book is informed by the latest evidence-based research about funerals, the thick descriptions afforded by ethnography, and the best theoretical constructs of how the meaning-making function of bereavement operates. But its fundamental goal is to apply those ideas to practice in such a way that bereavement counselors, hospice professionals, funeral directors, clergy, and a host of volunteer caregivers provide more effective and compassionate care for bereaved individuals and families.

The volume regularly blends together terms like "funeral," "memorial ceremony," and "ritual," though each term has its own unique meaning. The U.S. Federal Trade Commission, for example, defines a funeral as a service with the body present and a memorial service as one without it. Nevertheless, both terms along with their more contemporary synonyms such as "celebration of life," "homegoing," and "memorial gathering" all attempt to label the varied ways humans begin making sense of death and their own experience with loss by enacting various kinds of memorial activities.

These memorial activities might be considerably broader than *the* funeral per se because they involve such communal activities as the Jewish custom of unveiling of the gravestone near the first anniversary of the death, the group of teenagers who work together on a temporary roadside memorial near the place their friend was killed, or the annual observances held more than two decades after the terrorist attacks of 9/11. Whether we would define these as "the funeral" or not, they are symbol-infused activities in which we attempt to create meaning when emotions seem uncontrollable and words fail us.

This volume begins with an overview of the theoretical concept I developed in clinical practice decades ago and have confirmed in my own research. Simply stated, I posit that there are several unique anchors that are predictably found throughout history and around the world in the ways people attempt to create meaning in the immediate aftermath of a death. Chapter 1 recaps those anchors—significant symbols, gathered community, ritual action, connection to heritage, and transition of the corpse—and applies them to a landscape that has changed over the decade since the concept was first published.

During the first years of my pastoral psychology career, I surmised that the people I was caring for did not proceed through bereavement in any stepwise, linear fashion in spite of the plethora of stage-based and phase-based models that dominated the bereavement landscape of the 1970s and 1980s. In listening to bereaved individuals, I began to hear their common descriptions of four adaptive actions they were taking on their grief journeys. Their quest seemed less about recovering from their loss than enfolding the experiences with loss into the remaining chapters of their lives in a process I came to eventually call *integrating the loss*. Chapter 2 explores the concept of meaning making in bereavement considering its relationship to these adaptive actions taken by bereaved people, not as steps on their journey but rather as ongoing elements of the rest of their lives as they continually tell stories, find meanings, face the realities of the loss, and say goodbye to their loved ones.

Anyone working with the dying and bereaved has undoubtedly noticed that much of what is done in the ceremonies of death grow out of the need to make meaning of what faith says in the face of loss. Chapter 3 explores the varied ways that religious faith and beliefs enter the conversation about funerals, how these beliefs bear directly on the memorial customs that families and communities observe, and how these customs sometimes get challenged by families divided along religious lines. Even though I am a person of faith—one whose own faith has been demonstrably tested by the deaths of two children before birth, a fatal car crash in which I was severely injured and that resulted in the deaths of two friends, and a host of others—this book is not a personal apologetic for the role of faith in crisis. Rather, this chapter looks at what the extant evidence indicates is the profoundly important role of religious faith in coping with crisis.

Although some have suggested the death of a child is "the biggest loss," this is a uniquely Western interpretation, often not shared in many parts of the developing world. Moreover, these words tend to minimize the losses in other types of death-related bereavement. Nevertheless, the death of a child or adolescent presents unique challenges to families and communities as they organize memorial gatherings in the face of such meaning disruption. These funerals seek to speak order into the chaos of a death so apparently "out of time," and they often must provide meaningful participation to a throng of classmates and other contemporaries of the deceased. How families and communities deal with a child's death and funeral is the topic explored in Chapter 4.

A favorite topic of media outlets since the 1970s has been the "high cost of dying" and yet, despite widespread consumer advocacy and reforms including government regulations in many jurisdictions, families and communities still "spend with abandon" when it comes to honoring their dead. One of the most perplexing dilemmas of all for development experts has been the largely unbending choice of bereaved families and communities to pursue cultural customs in death, even when doing so risks economic disaster, and in the case of the 2014 Ebola crisis in West Africa, even the health of the bereaved family and community. Sorting out these thorny issues against a backdrop of how families and communities create meaning is the topic of Chapter 5.

Although the experiences of loss are usually integrated into the mourner's life in healthy, adaptive ways, that is not always the case. The precursor to such complicated grief is often bound up with the circumstances of the death (trauma and violence), with a lack of support to the bereaved, or with some underlying issue that long predated the experience with loss. The ways such complexities affect memorial ceremonies and when and how memorial ceremonies might be beneficial to prevent these clinically complicated experiences are the subject of Chapter 6. When bereavement gets complicated, perhaps even leading to what can clinically be defined as prolonged grief disorder, therapeutic rituals can be beneficial.

When the COVID-19 pandemic struck in the early months of 2020, no one could have imagined its impact on the physical health, economy, and mental well-being of the world's inhabitants. No one from the most advanced city to the village of a developing nation would escape the ravages of the disease or the effects—of both the disease and the social and governmental policies enacted to stop its spread. Because of their tendency to gather large groups of people, funerals were among the first activities altered by government lockdowns and quarantines. Chapter 7 explores how these social policies changed the ways funerals were conducted in the moment and discusses the already-emerging research about what the long-term impacts of these changes may be on bereaved families and communities.

Much of what has been discussed in the first seven chapters—the ubiquity of the anchors, the quest to create meaning, the dependence on spiritual resources in the face of loss, funerals for and including children, the economic challenges of funeral options in a setting of low resources, the challenges of complicated grief from trauma, and the vagaries of the pandemic—all come together in the extended case analysis of funeral ceremonies among African Americans explored in Chapter 8. These "homegoings," as they are often called, are ceremonies designed to honor the life and legacy of the deceased while providing comfort and solace for family, friends, and the community at large.

This book does not intend to be the final word on memorial ceremonies. There will undoubtedly be many changes and challenges ahead as humans seek to find culturally appropriate, spiritually fulfilling, and emotionally effective ways to mourn the loss of a loved one. Chapter 9 acknowledges that the work has just begun amid a plethora of funeral adaptations as bereaved individuals, families, and communities seek to create meaning in loss through their death ceremonies. The newer innovations related to death and grief—human composting, alkaline hydrolysis, rental caskets for cremation, a return to natural burial, memorial jewelry, and nonprofit funeral providers—are all attempts to help people find greater meaning in the ceremonies so that the grief process gets started well. Where humans have been in death ceremonies and where groups seem to be headed next is the subject of the final chapter of this book.

This volume's epilogue is an intensely personal reflection on two recent funerals in my own family. As I walked with my brother's family through his death in 2021 and that of his son 14 months earlier, I realized afresh how important this gathering together in the face of death is for the human family. We derive support from rubbing shoulders and sharing tears with family and friends against the backdrop of storytelling and faith rekindling. After four decades walking alongside families like my own, I attest again that these observances are invaluable in helping families and communities in the arduous process of *creating meaning in funerals*.

Reference

Popovsky, M.A. (2007, May). *Jewish ritual, reality, and response at the end of life: A guide to caring for Jewish patients and their families*. Duke Institute on Care at the End of Life/Duke Divinity School. https://www.iceol.duke.edu.

Chapter 1

Anchors of Ceremony

How Funerals Work

Imagine a funeral for David, a "child of the Depression," born in 1924 who never really escaped the "frugal ways" of growing up in that period. His childhood was marked by sadness and deprivation. His father died when David was only eight and so he left high school as a 15-year-old to help pay for the family's expenses. After serving four years in World War II, he married the "girl of his dreams," and together they reared five children in their quiet town. Even though David neither finished high school nor went to college, he was a lifelong learner and he never quit finding new ways to make the most of the automobile repair business he opened and grew throughout his adult life. When he retired at age 69, he and his wife had amassed a large enough nest egg to travel, fund their grandchildren's education, and enjoy the purchase of a new car every few years.

David was a man of quiet faith, but he and his beloved Sally sat together every week in the pews of the town's Baptist church where they had been married, reared their children, and worshipped. So it was altogether fitting, Sally thought, that when David died of a massive heart attack at the age of 87, his funeral should be held on that early autumn Wednesday morning in the same small church where they had devoted their lives for more than 65 years of marriage. The visitation at the funeral home on Tuesday evening brought the entire community together; congregants, neighbors, friends, and former customers stopped in to pay their respects, share their stories, and honor the life of "the best mechanic this county's ever seen," the president of the town bank said to David's oldest son.

Some people made charitable contributions in David's honor. However, more than 25 individuals and organizations ignored the suggestion of donations to charity and sent floral arrangements of every size, shape, and color to the funeral home. David took pride in his own rose garden, and the town florist was able to utilize about 40 of David's own roses in the flower arrangement that sat atop the polished walnut casket. On a table near the casket the funeral director had arranged a few of David's tools, a couple of older auto repair manuals, and some photos taken over the years at the shop. A folded American flag was positioned in the casket just

DOI: 10.4324/9781003353010-2

behind David's head and his hands were folded around his study Bible from which he had read and learned for nearly 50 years.

The funeral service at the Baptist church was exactly what David and Sally had talked about in recent years, filled with scripture and southern gospel music. The minister talked about David's faith and his hard work, his love of family and community, and his never-ending willingness to help someone in need. The pastor acknowledged the pain of loss, never minimizing the struggles Sally would face as she learned to adjust to a life without David, and he suggested practical actions members of the community could take in coming alongside Sally. The pastor also explained the reason for Sally's hope in the face of her beloved's death: "Sally knows without a doubt that David knew where he was headed. Because of the choice to follow Jesus he made when he was just a boy and that commitment lived out throughout his life," the pastor explained, "we don't have to worry about David. He is safe in the arms of Jesus, ready to take up his eternal residence in the mansion prepared for him."

The pastor's words seemed especially poignant as the church's pianist and a lone vocalist began their own arrangement of blind, 19th-century hymnist Fanny Crosby's "Safe in the arms of Jesus, / Safe on His gentle breast, / There by His love o'ershaded, / Sweetly my soul shall rest" (Crosby, 1868).

When the last prayers had been offered, the final hymns of faith sung, and the family had taken its time to say a final goodbye to David's body, the funeral director, with the help of David's children, solemnly closed the casket, led the mourners out of the church to the waiting hearse, and finally, drove David the "last mile of the way" to the town cemetery just a few blocks away. Rather than drive the most direct route from church to cemetery in leading the procession, the funeral director detoured to the north, taking mourners on a route that passed the shop where David had repaired hundreds of cars for his neighbors and friends. Upon reaching the business, the funeral director paused for a few moments to allow family and friends to reflect on the meaning of this location they all knew so well and that symbolized the man's life so completely.

Although a composite of several funerals, the details of David's life and funeral provide a highly accurate picture of the way many funerals are conducted, especially in southern and midwestern towns of the United States. Even as cremation has grown in popularity and "simple memorial services" have become more commonplace than they were a few decades ago, the so-called traditional funeral is anything but dead in many places and for many families.

In a bygone era, funerals could be expected to follow an almost cookie-cutter model, depending on whether the deceased was Jewish, Catholic, or Southern Baptist. Today's "traditional funeral," however, like David's service, is far more likely to include personalized symbols and even ceremonies that relate to the specific details of his life, his work, and his faith. In interviews for this book, one responding funeral director with more than 40 years of experience referred to his work as similar to that of a wedding planner where no detail is too small to be considered. He then quipped, "The only problem is, we have three days to organize all the details."

This funeral director's mention of the short time available to plan is significant. From time immemorial, social groups have closely attached the initial memorial rituals to the early mourning period, often creating funeral gatherings within hours or certainly no more than a few days after the death. During the Middle Ages, European Christians often planned the funeral ceremonies of their loved ones to occur on the third day following death, a salute to the Christian belief that Jesus arose from the grave on the third day. The third-day sentiment has followed many older believers into their 21st-century lives. In both Islam and Judaism, funerals traditionally occur before sundown on the day of death and no later than the day after.

Sometimes traditionally religious, sometimes intensely personal and poignant, and most often, some combination of these, funeral ceremonies help bereaved individuals and families create meaning in the face of a death—whether that loss was long expected or traumatic. Anthropologists have long recognized the value of these life transition rituals that assist the bereaved in navigating the leave-taking from their dead and the putting on of a new post-bereavement identity across the chasm of an indeterminate "betwixt time" Van Gennep (1909/1960) called liminality. Funeral ceremonies are particularly helpful to the bereaved because in so many emotional ways, especially when death came unexpectedly, the dead are not yet fully apprised to be dead for the mourners who are left behind (Kastenbaum, 2004).

In this volume's predecessor, *Do Funerals Matter? The Purposes and Practices of Death Rituals in Global Perspective* (Hoy, 2013), readers were introduced to a process of thinking about memorial ceremonies around the world and throughout history through the lens of five anchors. Like ceremonies planned by families and communities around the globe and throughout history, in extraordinarily meaningful ways, the funeral David's family arranged with the help of their funeral director and pastor addressed all five of these anchors. That earlier book theorized that these five anchors are virtually universal in their application. A decade later, this volume reaffirms the notion that significant symbols, gathered community, ritual action, connection to cultural heritage, and transition of the body work in concert to help individuals, families, and entire mourning communities create meaning in the face of death.

Significant Symbols

David's story, with which this chapter began, illustrates the role of significant symbols. The solid walnut casket in David's story would possibly have reminded his wife and children of the furniture that graces so many southern homes of their generation. Perhaps his wife thought that although he never spent much money on himself, David's love for "fine furniture" justified the purchase even though most funeral homes display caskets in a wide range of prices. Caskets constructed from finely crafted hardwoods like walnut, cherry, and maple are typically priced well above the median among any funeral provider's options.

Interestingly, during the early writing of this manuscript, our family arranged the funeral for Margaret Jean Coffey (1932–2022), my wife's mother. More than 25 years earlier when she and Debbie's dad visited us in Southern California, the two of them showed us the caskets they would select for themselves. Although the unit my father-in-law chose was no longer available when he died in 2016, the Batesville Laurel Maple Margaret had chosen was a special-order item obtainable by the funeral home serving us when she died. I never asked her what attracted her to the highly polished maple, but it undoubtedly reminded her of the Early American maple with which her own living room was furnished. Most likely, the same "taste" that caused her to choose her living room furniture figured into her choice of a casket as well. As such, it represented an important symbol for her family, if for no other reason than that it had been *her* choice. Considerations about cost (which was considerable) did not even enter our family's conversation.

Our family's experience selecting Margaret's casket is not unusual. After a brief introduction to available options, families arranging funerals in funeral establishments are generally left alone to make their selectin in private, away from possible selling interference from staff. Many expensive caskets exist with a high level of "eye appeal." And yet, in interviews with families and observation in funeral homes, I have rarely noted families opting for the least expensive option displayed. Both in my own family and in the dozens I have accompanied in this process, I cannot recall a single instance in which the least expensive casket was selected. In accompanying my brother's wife and their adult children to make funeral arrangements when he died in 2021, the family gravitated to a highly polished hardwood with exquisite detail in part because, as his son described, "Dad loved his woodworking [hobby] so much."

In David's story, the deeply customized flower arrangement, which included specimens from his own garden is an example of ways families have employed their loved one's hobbies in the symbolic parts of the memorial ceremonies. Funeral directors and bereaved family members alike describe the collections of dolls, garden tools, and books that are often part of the display near the casket or urn or elsewhere in the room. Motorcycles, cases of beer, and substantial libraries of classic books are just a few of the memorabilia displays I have seen.

One interview respondent explained the value of her family gathered around the dining room table selecting photographs for the video montage. Many funeral directors have echoed her sentiment that the process of storytelling that occurs in this photo selection may be more helpful than the photos themselves. In every case, these symbols utilized by mourners tell stories and communicate meanings in rich ways about life, character, and faith. *Life symbols* are the pictures mourners employ to remind each other of the life that their loved one lived. David's tools, auto repair manual, Bible, and roses from his garden all told stories about the important elements of David's life.

Mourners have used such symbols as far back as history is recorded. Grave goods excavated from the Seine Valley of France dating to more than 6,600 years ago show evidence of arrowheads and shells buried with the deceased (Hoy, 2013; Thomas et al., 2011) while cemeteries from the same region and Middle Neolithic Period (ca. 4700–3500 BCE) feature grave monuments of immense size and striking detail (Cheung et al., 2021).

Likewise, flowers are not a recent contribution to funeral rituals; archaeological evidence indicates the use of flora millennia ago. Mégaloudi and colleagues (2007), for example, discovered pomegranate and grape seeds in the northern Greek necropolis of Limenas, leading these archaeologists to conclude that the plants were interred with bodies, likely as part of religious rites surrounding death. Moreover, at the same site dating to the fourth century BCE, the researchers found 18 whole cloves of garlic ranging in size from 15 mm to 19 mm. The researchers noted that the size of the cloves indicate the likelihood they were cultivated rather than having grown randomly in the natural environment.

Along with myriad other religiously significant symbols, the personal Bible displayed in the deceased's hands, like David's in the story with which this chapter began, is a familiar symbolic way that bereaved individuals create meaning through funeral ceremonies. The reading of scripture and other sacred writings, the playing and singing of religious music, and the adorning of funeral chapels or worship spaces with religious symbols such as crosses, crucifixes, and Stars of David all speak to the importance of faith symbols in ceremonies.

Both the white funeral pall covering the casket to recall the deceased's baptism and the incensing of the body in the final commendation of the Roman Catholic funeral speak to the role of faith symbols in some liturgical contexts. Among some traditional Jews living outside of Israel, there is a deep desire to have a small amount of Israeli soil placed under the head of the deceased in the coffin before it is closed. Because of its deep religious meanings, fragrant sandalwood and its oil is vital in Hindu life-cycle rituals, not only at death but also at the birth of new family members (Rajendran, 2019). Each of the 12 traditional clans of the Hmong of the Laotian highlands has its own preferred tree for the use of burial coffins, and to use the wood from the wrong clan is to consign the dead to wander among the wrong people in the afterlife. Clearly, symbols matter to families and communities arranging mourning rituals.

In the research undergirding this volume, I found some bereaved survivors describing great efforts to create contemporary memorial events that would be devoid of religious meanings, ancient tradition, and tired ritual. Perhaps the choice of terms like "celebration of life" are even, at least in part, intended to signal something new in the way life is commemorated.

Nevertheless, these same individuals often employ such symbols as candles, music, and flowers, likely unaware they are following a long heritage of tradition in the use of these items and that these traditions often have religious foundations. One bereaved adult daughter, for example, described the painstaking efforts employed to persuade the city to permit the planting of a memorial tree accompanied by an engraved bronze plaque in her father's memory in a city park. According to her, municipal authorities did not like her idea because it was so innovative. As she described the high value she and her family placed on this rich symbol, she seemed unaware that her family was actually upholding a tradition that could be dated to the Middle Neolithic period, at least 5,500 years earlier.

Gathered Community

Around the world and throughout history, humans have tended to gather with one another in the face of tragedy. One of the most difficult parts of the COVID-19 global pandemic was the isolation that grew out of restrictions on social gathering, complicating the bereavement of many people who were already struggling with loneliness and isolation. Although this topic is addressed in more detail in Chapter 3 of this volume, it is important to note here as well because nowhere is humans' need for community more evident than in their behavior in the wake of a loved one's death.

In virtually every society studied, when notification of a death is received, family and friends go immediately to the side of those most closely bereaved. There is something humanly instinctive about our need to gather in the face of tragedy, a fact widely reported in the days following the 9/11 terrorist attacks in 2001 when complete strangers embraced and gathered in solidarity and mourning.

The gathering of people in the face of loss is well documented in the sociological literature on crowd behavior. Scholars such as Goode (1992, p. 181) have observed that in the face of traumatic circumstances, for example, crowd participants work together to define and find solutions to problems, usually responding to the chaos of tragedy with calm resolve and thoughtfulness rather than with panic.

Reflecting on her coverage of New York Catholic priest and fire chaplain Mychal Judge's funeral on September 15, 2001 at Saint Francis of Assisi Church, *New York Times* photographer Suzanne DeChillo (2021) noted her initial disappointment at not being able to get into the church to photograph the event. Instead, she walked across the street to the Engine 21/Ladder 1 firehouse where a large crowd had gathered. At the end of the homily for his friend, Fr. Michael Duffy instructed mourners to stand and hold out their hand to pronounce the benediction on their beloved Fr. Judge, and the photographer captured a photo of dozens in front of the firehouse following the same instruction given to mourners inside the church, joining in the solidarity of gathered community in the face of tragedy.

Walker and Balk (2007) tell of the importance of gathering for a wake on the night before the funeral for mourners of the Creek Nation in eastern Oklahoma. These gatherings, often lasting well into the night, typically include multiple speakers telling stories and honoring the life and character of the deceased. This example is repeated in community groups of diverse faith traditions, ethnic backgrounds, and geographic locations. Mourners need to both tell and hear stories, and this process can most clearly be accomplished in the context of a group.

The rhetoric of eulogies help to cement in the minds of mourners the character of the deceased and the valuable impact that person had on the world. After establishing one's credibility to deliver the eulogy, eulogizers tend to praise the deceased, disclose their own emotion, suggest actions for problem-focused coping, positively reappraise the death (i.e., make references to blissful afterlife), and affirm a continued relationship with the deceased, often by addressing the deceased directly (Dennis & Kunkel, 2004; Kunkel & Dennis, 2003).

Gathering together is vital because it creates solidarity with others who also hurt. The old adage that "grief shared is grief lessened" seems intuitively true, and humans seem nearly incapable of allowing their bereaved family members and friends to face crisis utterly alone, even when the bereaved might have wished for relished privacy.

Physical presence provides opportunity to bear witness to another's experience, even when there are no words that can ease the burden of the loss. Bereaved individuals rarely express a wish they had been left alone in their grief. Rather, these bereaved individuals most frequently report amazement so many people attended memorial ceremonies or simply stopped what they were doing to pay their respects for the dead and to bear witness with the mourners' suffering.

One bereaved father reported how overwhelmed he felt as he followed his son's casket into the church for the funeral mass. As he saw the throng of co-mourners, he immediately concluded that his son "really made an impact on the world . . . and we are not in this by ourselves" (Hoy, 2013, p. 52).

Ritual Action

In the earlier volume (Hoy, 2013), I titled the chapter on ritual action "Walk Out What You Can't Talk Out" (p. 66). Intuitively, bereaved individuals long to do something in the face of their sorrow and participating in rituals—whether prescribed by tradition or invented in the moment—seem to be just the needed remedy. When mourners "aid in burying" their dead or participate in other activities in the face of their grief, they are joining with ancestors in utilizing movement to manage emotion. Whether bathing the deceased, digging a grave, bearing the body to the tomb, kneeling in reverence, beating a drum, or preparing a salad to contribute to the "casserole caravan," getting busy in doing something is a natural human response to loss (Hoy, 2013, p. 66).

Within 90 minutes of my father's death, neighbors and church friends began to appear at the door of my mother's home, each bearing a casserole, cake, pie, salad, or other "comfort food." This tradition of bringing food is so much a part of the funeral landscape of the southern United States where my parents lived that people stopped what they were doing to attend to my family's needs even before we knew what those needs were. My family was immediately drawn back into the deep sense of caring on the part of that community evidenced by their simple acts of service. Only in later reflection, however, did I realize that in addition to serving an important need for our family, those community members were in effect also expressing their own grief at my father's death; the preparation and delivery of food was an important meaning-creating activity for them as they sought to express their own emotion of loss. Words did not come easily to most of those bringing food, but their practical action spoke volumes to us and provided a meaningful way for them to grieve with us.

Paxton (1990) noted the apparent unchanging human need for ritual:

> Rituals do things. They are performances, participatory activities that involve groups of people—people who learn things through their participation in rituals. They can model the way in which crisis or change has been met in the past and suggest ways to meet it in the future.
>
> (pp. 8–9)

In my fieldwork in Nyakach, Nyanza, Kenya from 2012 to 2017, I learned of the importance of community members "putting their back into" digging graves in the hard rocky soil so they can bury their community members. As many as 30 men of all ages join in the process of preparing the grave when a member of the community dies. The community role of digging the grave is not unique to sub-Saharan Africa; the tradition is still practiced in some rural American ranching and farming communities.

In a similar vein, Bliatout (1993) noted the wide variety of helpers who join in the process of creating funeral rituals when a member of the Hmong community dies. The Hmong originate in the hill country of Laos, Vietnam, and Thailand. After facing persecution in the early 1970s for being an ally of the United States during the Vietnam War, the Hmong began immigrating to the United States, settling especially in Wisconsin, Minnesota, and the central valley of California where sponsoring organizations first welcomed them. Funeral service professionals in these communities confirm that even among acculturated Hmong immigrants, there seems to be an expectation there will be many of the identified helpers for traditional funerals, including "guides" to the spirit world, reed pipers, drummers, descendent counselors, funeral coordinators, food servers, chefs, burial garment makers, and many others (Bliatout, 1993, pp. 86–88). In addition to the spiritual role these helpers play in assisting the deceased's spirit to the next world and the emotional comfort these caregiving tasks undoubtedly are to families, these helpers are likely actualizing their own experiences with communal grief through their participation in these rituals.

Thousands of people stood on the street outside the Newark, New Jersey church where songwriter and recording artist Whitney Houston's funeral was being held. Even though some people had driven many miles and waited for hours on the street, their simple presence with others in solidarity, bearing witness to the collective grief, seemed essential to their own well-being. We have witnessed such communal grieving every time a person of fame dies and often even the funerals of those unknown in life but made celebrities by their deaths, such as George Floyd. Both funerals are discussed more fully in Chapter 8 of this volume.

Whether a community responds to a person's death by bringing food to the bereaved home, by participating in digging the grave, by serving as a pallbearer, or by joining in a community process of wailing, participation in the action of ritual seems to be vital for mourners, both in the immediate circle of bereaved persons and in the wider community.

Connection to Cultural Heritage

While some pundits suggest that funeral rituals have been significantly upended by cultural shifts, at least when viewed through the prism of these five anchors, memorial rituals tend to change at a glacially slow pace. Elements of ceremony with ancient roots—such as fire, earth, water, and air—are still utilized in contemporary funeral rituals around the world.

Although subject in some places to the same pressures being exerted on other traditional mourning practices, Roman Catholic rituals in most parishes around the world place significant emphasis on the connection to cultural heritage that is embedded in this faith community's theology and practices. There are undoubtedly deep theological reasons for the prescribed rituals of this faith community, but the predictability of the rites seems to be part of what actually speaks calm into the chaos of early grief (Kellehear, 2007).

The *Order of Christian Funerals*, the prescribed liturgy for funerals in the Roman Catholic Church throughout the English-speaking world, as well as its translation into Spanish (*El ritual de exequias Cristianas*) provides a multiphase order to funeral ceremonies. Catholic funerals conducted in languages other than English or Spanish follow the approved Latin version, *Ordo exsequiarium*. Roman Catholic funeral liturgies are not designed as do-it-yourself affairs with broad opportunities to deviate from the prescribed rites. In the traditional multisegment funeral, a vigil service, usually held the night before the funeral mass, is a time of gathering for family and friends to offer prayers, read scripture, and share stories. This ceremony is where most eulogizing and formal storytelling occurs in Roman Catholic funerals.

The funeral mass or liturgy itself, generally held in the deceased's own parish church, begins with the reception of the body, the sprinkling of the casket with water taken directly from the baptismal font, and in most cases, the placing of a white linen pall on the casket to recall the deceased's own baptism shortly after birth. Clergy and altar servers bearing the symbols of the faith—a crucifix, a candle, and the printed Book of the Gospels—precede the casket and family in a deliberate processional journey down the church's center aisle toward the altar, reminiscent of the deceased's own journey of faith observed throughout his or her life. The music that is sung, the scriptures that are read, the homily that is delivered, and the eucharistic meal that is shared by the gathered mourners all point to the deceased person's life of faith. Then, at the culmination of the mass, the body is traditionally incensed by the priest in a custom that is both ancient and pregnant with meaning as mourners imagine the rising smoke as a symbol of their own prayers rising toward heaven.

After departing the church and frequently traveling in an automobile or walking procession to the cemetery, family and friends bid farewell to the deceased, leaving the mortal remains in the cemetery so that mourners can get back to the business of living their lives (Canine, 1996). Finally, the traditional Roman Catholic funeral liturgy culminates in the prayers of blessing and gratitude offered at the grave or the crematorium. Although language has been updated by the occasional changing of a word here and a phrase there, these rites have not been substantially tampered with in centuries. A Roman Catholic believer from the medieval period would likely recognize many of the ceremonial elements present in a 21st-century Roman Catholic funeral.

This slow pace of change is likely explained by the tendency of cultural groups to maintain life-cycle ritual observances long after otherwise assimilating into a new culture. Ceremonies of birth, coming of age (puberty), marriage, and death are seemingly characterized by common factors long after other cultural practices and even language fade from common use.

One funeral director reported his observation that although more than 35% of the bereaved families served say they are not religious, when shown a book with a wide variety of suggested verse for the memorial folder, these same families overwhelmingly select Psalm 23 for the folder. Even if they do not espouse connection to a faith community, if this funeral director's report is to be believed, many of his families find comfort in the trusted words of faith that begin, "The Lord is my shepherd, I shall not want" (Psalm 23:1 AV).

Transition of the Body

In both his writing and recorded interviews, Michigan funeral director and early 21st-century "spokesman" for the funeral service profession Thomas Lynch has observed the importance of the body at funerals. Lynch noted that among some contemporary people groups, the presence of the dead at the funeral has "become optional." He stated,

> That is probably not good for the culture at large. Up until a couple of generations ago, humans dealt with death by dealing with their dead so the way we *processed mortality* was by *processing from one place to the other*. And both the dead and the living have some distance to go when someone we love dies.
>
> (Navasky & O'Connor, 2007, loc. 03:50–04:40)

One of the pioneers of the pastoral counseling movement noted a half century ago that religious groups that were more "rationalistic" in their orientation to faith were working to reduce or eliminate ritual from their worship practices. These groups, he explained, "sought to develop a tradition largely without ceremony and substituted a direct appeal to the intellect." He went on to hypothesize that their growth had been thwarted, at least in part, because of their failure "to recognize the emotional needs that were being satisfied by the opportunities for acting out" (Jackson, 1975, p. 24).

From time immemorial and across cultures, funeral ceremonies have been fundamentally linked with the removal of the corpse from society. The necessity of moving the dead physical remains to a permanent place of repose has had both emotional and practical foundations. Van Gennep (1909/1960) noted the importance of this corpse transition more than a century ago and described multiple examples of highly ritualized, deeply symbolic, and extraordinarily elaborate rites of transition. Among his thick cultural descriptions was an extensive explanation of the 16-step process followed by the Kol, one of the largest people groups in India, to take care of the corpse between death and final committal of the cremated remains. The traditional ceremonies included painting the color yellow onto the corpse to ward off evil spirits, processing along a circuitous route, scattering rice along the procession route so that a returning spirit would not bother neighbors, and sharing ceremonial meals. These acts, along with many other rites of separation that Van Gennep noted, were often far more complex than any other aspect of funeral ceremonies. Finally, among the Kol, a type of betrothal ceremony was traditionally held at which wedding music was performed as the deceased's cremated remains were united (in marriage) with the spirits of the lower world (Van Gennep, 1909/1960, pp. 151–152).

Van Gennep (1909/1960) and other anthropologists have long been intrigued by the importance placed on the removal of the body from the place of the living to its permanent home in the "abode of the dead" (p. 146). Often, this ceremonial transition of the corpse was seen as necessary to prevent a restless spirit from bothering the living relatives and friends of the deceased. Prothero (2001) noted that death changes a living being into a corpse and this "new thing," the corpse, "represents, among other things, a threat to social order, an economic burden to the family, a reminder of our mortality, an offense to sight and smell, an affront to hopes of eternal life, and a reason to believe in the bodily resurrection" (p. 1).

Contemporary, industrialized, urban Westerners might balk at such concepts, but in my own experience, I have seen no expense spared by governments, families, and other parties to reclaim dead bodies after transportation accidents. In her work regarding the difficulty of ambiguous loss, Boss (2002) suggested there is a basic "primitive need" to be in the presence of the remains so that one can separate from the individual who has died. She affirmed the importance of the dead body, suggesting that "paradoxically, *having* the body enables [bereaved individuals] to let go of it" (p. 15). Boss told of a family who upon realizing they had no body to bury, rented a coffin and put the dead man's guitar in it for the funeral, buried the guitar, and finally, returned the coffin.

Recovery of remains from the 1999 crash of the airplane piloted by John F. Kennedy Jr., son of the assassinated president, were estimated to have far exceeded US$500,000 (CBS News, 1999). Ironically, after recovery, the bodies of Kennedy, his wife, and his sister-in-law were cremated and the remains scattered back in the ocean three miles from the site of the crash from which the bodies were initially recovered 24 hours earlier (MacQuarrie, 1999). Especially when death has been by traumatic circumstances, there seems to be an important need to recover the remains before allowing for the transition to the body's more permanent "home."

The only bodies that seem to be on "permanent display," in fact, are those that are assigned a virtually divine nature to be revered and worshipped by an adoring public. Such is the case with the body of Soviet founder Vladimir Lenin, whose body was painstakingly embalmed by two pathologists shortly after his death in 1924 and has remained on near continuous display to the public ever since (Milton, 2015).

Thought by some to be a unique American custom, the viewing of the corpse has been found in several studies to have beneficial effects for mourners. Harrington and Sprowl (2011) conducted in-depth interviews with 16 Canadian individuals bereaved by the sudden death of a loved one, finding that all but one respondent had an "instinctual need or drive to view" (p. 75). Interestingly, participants expressed appreciation for multiple opportunities to view the body at the scene, hospital, and funeral home, even when the loved person had been disfigured by an accident or suicide. The researchers found that many of their respondents sensed a need to take care of their family member, especially during the early hours of transition from life to death. In a particularly poignant anecdote, a mother recounted that she was told at the scene of her son's death in a car crash that he had died instantly. Nevertheless, she explained, she regretted that she had not held her son "one last time," wondering aloud, "Maybe he was still there inside . . . waiting for me, waiting for his mother to just come by and hold him" (p. 76).

Similarly, some pediatric hospices in the United Kingdom have begun using special cooling mattresses and rooms with abnormally low temperatures, described collectively as "cooling facilities" to retard decomposition, allowing parents and families to spend time with their deceased child. Hackett and colleagues (2022) found that among 30 parents interviewed, all were grateful for the opportunity, describing the process as helpful in allowing them to make the transition from caring for their child to acknowledging the child's death. All respondents believed the opportunity should be available to all parents following a child's death, indicating they treasured the time with their child.

Although it seems trite, societies throughout history have not allowed the dead to lie where they fall, rather preferring to move them from the place of the living to a more permanent abode in the place of the dead (Canine, 1996).There seems to be an instinctual emotional need to move the dead, but the removal of the corpse from the community also serves a practical purpose. Decomposing flesh is highly objectionable to the senses of most people, and the sights and smells as the body changes from living family member to inanimate corpse simply seems to be more than most people want to embrace.

Clinical Implications

In the years since *Do Funerals Matter?* (Hoy, 2013) was published, clergy, funeral directors, memorial celebrants, and other ritual leaders have affirmed the five anchors as a blueprint for creating meaningful ceremonies. A New York funeral home owner had a poster developed and mounted on the wall of his arrangement rooms that show the five anchors in the shape of a pyramid. The poster is intended to help families visually as they craft memorial ceremonies. One celebrant recently remarked, "When I sit with a family to begin creating a funeral ceremony, I have the five anchors in my mind and they guide the questions I ask. Later, as I am crafting the ceremony, those same five ideas become the cornerstone for what I do, what I say, how I lead."

Clinicians will want to inquire about memorial ceremonies in which the bereaved have participated. Through these interactions, it may be possible to discern parts of the ceremony that were omitted. Although it seems ideal that all five anchors are incorporated in the ceremonies around the time of the death, bereavement counselors can incorporate one or more of the anchors into therapeutic rituals to potentially help individuals and groups resolve complex experiences with bereavement (Castle & Phillips, 2003; Doka, 2002).

Whether a family or community group intentionally employs the five anchors thus described, however, it seems relatively instinctual that they will include these elements in the planning of memorial rituals. Whether a bereaved family employs a highly prescribed ritual, a personalized free-form memorial ceremony, or something in between, their choices seem driven intuitively by the need to begin creating meaning of the life and the death of the individual. Across the globe, funeral ceremonies give shape to the early bereavement process because they help provide form and calm to a chaotic experience.

Reflection and Discussion

- When you attend a funeral or memorial ceremony, what do you expect to see and experience? Does that usually happen?
- What would you want to make sure was included if you were planning your own memorial service?

- When you last attended a funeral that "failed miserably" for you, what happened? How would you have changed what was done to have made the ceremony more meaningful?
- Are you convinced by the author's premise that symbols, gathered community, ritual activities, connection to heritage, and transition of the body contribute to helping bereaved people create meaning in their loss? Why or why not?

References

Bliatout, B.T. (1993). Hmong death customs: Traditional and acculturated. In D.P. Irish, K.F. Lundquist, & V.J. Nelsen (Eds.), *Ethnic variations in dying, death, and grief: Diversity in universality* (pp. 79–100). Taylor & Francis.

Boss, P.G. (2002). Ambiguous loss: Working with families of the missing. *Family Process*, 41, 14–17.

Canine, J.D. (1996). *The psychosocial aspects of death and dying*. Appleton & Lange.

Castle, J., & Phillips, W.L. (2003). Grief rituals: Aspects that facilitate adjustment to bereavement. *Journal of Loss and Trauma*, 8, 41–71.

CBS News. (1999, August 4). JFK Jr. search cost $500K. https://www.cbsnews.com/news/jfk-jr-search-cost-500k/.

Cheung, C., Herrscher, E., Andre, G., Bedault, L., Hachem, L., Binois-Roman, A., Simonin, D., & Thomas, A. (2021). The grandeur of death: Monuments, societies, and diets in Middle Neolithic Paris Basin. *Journal of Anthropological Archaeology*, 63, 101332. https://doi.org/10.1016/j.jaa.2021.101332.

Crosby, F.J. (1868). Safe in the arms of Jesus [hymn text]. https://hymnary.org.

DeChillo, S. (2021, September 11). With bowed heads, American reflect on 9/11 and its aftermath. *New York Times*. https://www.nytimes.com/live/2021/09/11/nyregion/9-11-20th-anniversary.

Dennis, M.R., & Kunkel, A.D. (2004). Fallen heroes, lifted hearts: Consolation in contemporary presidential eulogia. *Death Studies*, 28(8), 703–731. https://doi.org/10.1080/07481180490483373.

Doka, K.J. (2002). The role of ritual in the treatment of disenfranchised grief. In K. J. Doka (Ed.), *Disenfranchised grief: New directions, challenges and strategies for practice* (pp. 135–147). Research Press.

Goode, E. (1992). *Collective behavior*. Harcourt Brace Jovanovich.

Hackett, J., Heavy, E., & Beresford, B. (2022). "It was like an airbag, it cushioned the blow": A multi-site qualitative study of bereaved parents' experiences of using cooling facilities. *Palliative Medicine*, 36(2), 365–374. https://doi.org/10.1177/02692163211059345.

Harrington, C., & Sprowl, B. (2011). Family members' experiences with viewing in the wake of sudden death. *Omega: Journal of Death and Dying*, 64(1), 65–82. https://doi.org/10.2190/OM.64.1.e.

Hoy, W.G. (2013). *Do funerals matter? The purposes and practices of death rituals in global perspective*. Routledge.

Jackson, E.N. (1975). *Parish counseling*. Jason Aronson.

Kastenbaum, R. (2004). Why funerals? *Generations*, 28(2), 5–10.

Kellehear, A. (2007). *A social history of dying*. Cambridge University Press.

Kunkel, A.D., & Dennis, M.R. (2003). Grief consolation in eulogy rhetoric: An integrative framework. *Death Studies*, 27(1), 1–38. https://doi.org/10.1080/07481180302872.

MacQuarrie, B. (1999, July 23). Kennedy, Bessette ashes cast from ship. *Boston Globe*. https://archive.boston.com/news/packages/jfkjr/0722_ashes.htm.

McClatchey, I.S., King, S., & Domby, E. (2021). From grieving to giving: When former bereavement campers return as volunteers. *Omega: Journal of Death and Dying*, 84(1), 228–244. https://doi.org/10.1177/0030222819886734.

Mégaloudi, F., Papadopoulos, S., & Sgourou, M. (2007). Plant offerings from the classical necropolis of Limenas, Thasos, northern Greece. *Antiquity*, 81(314), 933–943. https://doi.org/10.1017/S0003598X00096010.

Milton, G. (2015). *When Lenin lost his brain: Fascinating footnotes from history*. John Murray/Hachette.

Navasky, M., & O'Connor, K. (Writers and Producers). (2007, October 30). The undertaking (Episode 13) [TV series episode]. *PBS Frontline*. https://www.pbs.org/video/frontline-the-undertaking/.

Paxton, F.S. (1990). *Christianizing death: The creation of a ritual process in early medieval Europe*. Cornell University Press.

Prothero, S. (2001). *Purified by fire: A History of cremation in America*. University of California Press. https://doi.org/10.1525/j.ctt1pnnhg.

Rajendran, A. (2019, April 24). Chandan in Hinduism: Importance of sandalwood in Hindu religion. *Hindu Blog*. https://www.hindu-blog.com/2019/04/chandan-in-hinduism-importance-of.html.

Thomas, A., Chambon, P., & Murail, P. (2011). Unpacking burial and rank: The role of children in the first monumental cemeteries of Western Europe (4600–4300 BC). *Antiquity*, 85(329), 772–786. https://doi.org/10.1017/S0003598X00068307.

Van Gennep, A. (1960). *The rites of passage*. Translated by M.B. Vizedom & G.L. Caffee. University of Chicago Press. (Original work published 1909)

Walker, A.C., & Balk, D.E. (2007). Bereavement rituals in the Muskogee Creek tribe. *Death Studies*, 31, 633–652. https://doi.org/10.1080/07481180701405188.

Chapter 2

Funeral Ceremonies and the Quest for Meaning

When Miriam's husband died, nothing prepared her for the experience of his death or the days that followed. Married for nearly 38 years, Simon was "the picture of health," golfing, gardening, and jogging almost every day. Although there had been some history of heart disease in his family, Simon had avoided cigarettes and alcohol, the two substances he had long figured had led to his father's and brother's early deaths from heart disease. Simon ate a healthy diet and kept his stress level under wraps.

He awakened early that Tuesday morning, complaining of a tightness in his chest. When it did not abate, he got in the shower, thinking surely he had pulled a muscle working in his garden the day before. Miriam heard the crash, found him on the floor of their bathroom, and quickly summoned paramedics, but it was simply too late. Simon had died from what the autopsy report declared as "near complete occlusion of the anterior descending artery," the so-called widow maker. The death certificate showed that the "duration" from onset of his cardiac arrest to death was nearly "instantaneous."

Miriam's sister and brother-in-law were there within the hour, and Miriam and Simon's adult children arrived from their homes in other cities before that eventful day ended. Their community of friends surrounded them including Simon's work colleagues and their spouses, golf buddies, and friends from their temple including the young rabbi who had arrived in their community just a few months earlier. That initial support, Miriam would later report, was what buoyed her in those first hours after Simon's sudden death. But as she would say to her rabbi and to anyone else in earshot, what she could not figure out was how to make sense of this experience. Some folks cautioned, even on that first day in the midst of Miriam's questions, that "these things take time." Somehow, Miriam found even their attempted words of comfort to be of little help. The rituals of their faith—the communal funeral and burial, the shiva with the minyan leading the kaddish each evening—buoyed her sprits and provided direction in the chaos. But what she really wanted to know was, "Why now? Why him?"

DOI: 10.4324/9781003353010-3

Neimeyer (2019) has noted that the "central process in grieving is the attempt to reaffirm or reconstruct a world of meaning that has been challenged by loss" (p. 80), a point he has been making for years (Neimeyer, 2001). Moreover, much of the research in bereavement in recent years has focused on the role of meaning making. In one qualitative study, McClatchey and colleagues (2021) interviewed eight former bereavement camp participants who returned as young adults to guide the next generation of bereaved youngsters, finding a continuing sense of meaning in helping others.

For more than three decades, the pioneering work of Ronnie Janoff-Bulman (1992) has provided a theoretical foundation to the thoughts, questions, and emotions swirling in Miriam's head. She pointed out in her early research that humans live their lives in the context of an "assumptive world" and that loss, crisis, and trauma frequently "shatters" these assumptions. These inherent assumptions, Janoff-Bulman suggested, tend to revolve around our belief that the world is benevolent, that it is meaningful, and that we are worthy of the good that comes our way.

Wortman and Park (2009) have led the conversation that shattered assumptions are not necessarily inevitable. Some individuals derive deep meaning from spiritual and philosophical beliefs and they find the current loss tends to reaffirm those beliefs without significant challenge. In Park's (2005) initial presentation of a theory of how religion/spirituality (which she generally did not separate) as a tool of meaning making in adverse life circumstances, she asserted,

> While this work is ongoing, findings to date are unequivocal: Various aspects of religion are strongly related to physical and psychological well-being in everyday life in general, and in the context of coping with adversity in particular.
>
> (p. 707)

Gillies and Neimeyer (2006) argued a similar perspective in their meaning reconstruction model. They posit that a loved one's death either is or is not consistent with pre-loss meaning structures. If so, meaning is reaffirmed, and if not, distress increases. The bereaved individual's response to the increased distress, they suggested, is to attempt (1) sense making, (2) benefit finding, or (3) identity change. When one or more of these three strategies of the "search for meaning" are successful, Gillies and Neimeyer have suggested, the bereaved individual creates new meaning structures to accommodate the changes. If these discovered meanings are not helpful, they suggested, the process is cyclically repeated until new meanings are found that the individual can incorporate into the post-loss meaning structures (p. 55).

Yang and Lee (2022) summarized enumerable research studies to conclude that the evidence is compelling that a search for and subsequent discovery of meaning in loss leads to better overall grief adjustment, lower levels of mental health disorders such as anxiety and depression, improved physical health, increases in growth and self-esteem, more positive mood, and higher levels of life satisfaction. Nevertheless, clinicians and other caregivers often feel at a loss for how specifically to help bereaved individuals work through the process of creating meaning.

Road Signs on the Grief Journey: The Compass Model

Those who have attended one of my workshops on grief support and counseling might remember being asked to close their eyes and point to the north. For me, the exercise is always entertaining—as participants point in all possible directions. When those in attendance are invited to open their eyes and look around, they usually laugh at the diversity of responses—and the "directional challenge" with which most seem to be afflicted! In an unfamiliar room, one lacks the landmarks that help to "regain bearings." People quickly become disoriented and do not know which way is which. This activity provides an excellent picture of what it means to walk the journey called grief. The bereft person is lost in unfamiliar terrain, desperately needing *road signs*.

Integrating the Loss rather than Seeking Recovery

Now more than three decades in development (Hoy, 1993, 1996, 2007, 2016), the compass model grows out of a classic grounded theory research perspective (Glaser, 1998; Glaser & Strauss, 1967), directly resulting from clinical experience with hundreds of bereaved individuals and groups. This model assumes that the goal of the grief process is not *recovery* or *closure*, elusive terms at best. Rather, the goal of the meaning creation process of grief is that the bereaved person finds loss integrated into the rest of life. Major loss challenges the foundational set of beliefs about life's meaning and value; the integrational process of grief calls us to establish who we are now in the face of this loss and, perhaps more important, challenges bereaved individuals to inquire, "So what now?"

Whether settling frontiers or exploring new reaches of outer space, the greatest discoveries are preceded by a period in which the voyager is unsure where he or she is going, perhaps even a period of being completely lost. Whether navigating by the North Star or some familiar landmark, bereavement requires a stable, unchanging guide to find direction in grief. The image of a simple field compass with its needle pointing in the direction of north, south, east, or west is a metaphor that works for this purpose.

For most people, integrating the loss is a process undertaken naturally. We do not have to be told to "tell stories" or to "find meaning" or to "come to terms with the reality of the loss." These adaptive actions come rather naturally. They are not intended to be *prescriptive* but rather, *descriptive*. In other words, I am not suggesting how bereavement ought to progress as much as describing how it usually does proceed.

For most humans, the varied adjustment experiences following the death of a loved person are self-limiting. Our best evidence from multiple studies in the United States and elsewhere indicates perhaps only about 7% or so of all bereavements become "complicated" enough to meet any of a set of criteria for clinically significant and ongoing impairment in one's personal, work, social, or spiritual life (Bonanno, 2009; Shear, 2012). In other words, the vast majority of bereaved individuals "integrate" their losses into their lives with the support of family, community, friends, familiar rituals, and consideration (or renegotiation) of their belief systems. Moreover, in my experience, many complicated bereavement experiences can be diagnosed by seeing which of the directions on this compass are getting ignored in the adjustment to loss and then helping the bereaved individual to effectively address that road sign.

The bereavement caregiving community is relatively united that there are no such thing as "stages of grief" in terms of predictable, stepwise ways in which all or even most people approach loss. Although there are many similarities between individuals, there are few predictable "first this, then that, and then this other thing" in the grief process (Hoy, 2016; Worden, 2018). In a provocative paper, Stroebe and colleagues (2017) suggested that when health care professionals present stages as an operational model for grief, patients are poorly served:

> Major concerns include the absence of sound empirical evidence, conceptual clarity, or explanatory potential. It lacks practical utility for the design or allocation of treatment services, and it does not help identification of those at risk or with complications in the grieving process. Most disturbingly, the expectation that bereaved persons will, even should, go through stages of grieving can be harmful to those who do not.
>
> (pp. 455–456)

In conclusion, these eminent bereavement clinician-scholars said that stage theory should be discarded by professionals as well as by bereaved individuals themselves.

Unlike stages that logically must be addressed in sequence, these four adaptive actions—remembering, reaffirming, realizing, and releasing—work in concert to help the bereaved person, family, or community integrate this loss into the whole of life. As Figure 2.1 shows, these four road signs remind one where she or he is on the road to fully integrating this loss, "enfolding" the loss into the totality of a life that no longer includes the physical presence of the loved person who has died. Bereaved persons take specific actions to the extent of their emotional ability on each of these adaptations, revisiting them multiple times in the process of mourning. In my clinical work, I find bereaved people are often working

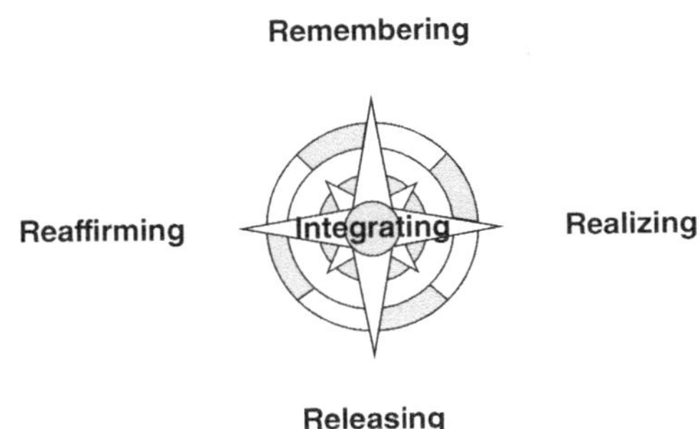

Figure 2.1 The Compass Model of Bereavement

on two or three of them simultaneously, and there is certainly no prescribed "progression" through stages.

When a loved one dies, we are faced with a series of choices that lead either to adaptation to a new way of living in a radically changed world or to grief that remains debilitating. The grief that is occasioned by a death-related loss is much more like an amputation to which one adapts than it is like a bad bruise or broken bone from which one fully recovers.

Nevertheless, some of the world's most powerful movements of change have occurred out of the context of a loss. Millions of dollars have been raised for cancer research and treatment because bereaved individuals started organizations to raise money and awareness. Mothers against Drunk Driving (MADD) was not started by a disinterested college student who decided to begin a nonprofit organization as a school project; this world-changing movement was begun by a bereaved California mother whose own teenaged daughter was killed at the hands of an impaired driver.

Parents whose teens and young adult children died by suicide have often been instrumental in creating foundations, funding research efforts, underwriting prevention programs, and acting as spokespersons for school assemblies to help others see the importance of early intervention. The vast majority of peer-led bereavement support groups are shepherded by individuals who have first lived through their own painful experiences of loss. All of these activities work in concert to help bereaved individuals integrate their experiences with loss.

Remembering

When families and communities engage in remembering a loved one's life, they recast his or her life and the relationship shared. Recalling the significant events, the funny stories, and the occasions when survival seemed to be a long shot all aid us in finding a place in life today for the relationship that has been disrupted by a death. But more than storytelling alone, these stories become the way in which we honor the values or character virtues that characterized the loved person's life.

One of the most helpful resources for people in grief is their memories. Bereavement groups, counselors who work with bereaved people, and friends of the bereaved help most when they provide plenty of time for people in grief to "tell their story," including the minute, mundane stories that make up a life and a relationship.

Recounting these memories usually evoke some mixture of joy and sadness. Tears are shed in telling even the funny stories and remembering the quirkiest of character qualities. In early grief, both pleasant and unpleasant memories are accompanied by sadness, but this unremitting sadness tends to abate for most people over time so that these memories are eventually recalled without the searing pain and sadness that is so commonplace in the early experience of loss.

Grief groups provide the opportunity for participants to share memories, stories, and photographs. Because other group members usually did not know each other's loved ones, they can hear the stories without correcting or supplementing.

However, in cultural groups around the world, the sharing of stories is a cardinal part of the funeral experience. Eulogies are packed with stories that are both poignant and humorous to the gathered mourners as the deceased's unique qualities and character are recalled. Photo collages, memorabilia collections, and life-tribute videos all provide a means to story sharing with a goal of honoring the character of the person who died, his or her faith and values, and the enduring impact he or she has made on the world. These stories become among the first means employed by bereaved family members and friends to create meaning of the loss, and funerals provide the culturally sanctioned way for these stories to be shared.

As important as the stories are, however, remembering is not just about storytelling; it is also about clarifying values. The stories shared by bereaved people point to the unique virtues that characterized the now-dead loved one. Generous, hardworking, patient, compassionate, joyful, peace loving, and teachable are just a few of the qualities that might have characterized this individual.

The meaning that is often found in a loved person's death turns on the "gifts" that individual imparted in the lives he or she touched. When bereaved people say, "This person changed my life," they usually mean, at least in part, "These are the characteristics of his or her life I will not only remember but perhaps even apply in my own life." Implicit in the sharing of stories is the honoring of the values that made this relationship truly valuable.

As important as sharing wonderful and pleasant memories is, caregivers must always remain mindful to the possibility that not all memories are pleasant. Funerals sometimes do—and often do not—acknowledge these real parts of life, but it is certainly possible that the deceased person's less savory character qualities could be brought out publicly in a funeral service. When such is the case, an important part of creating meaning in the story is wrestling with the stories of ambivalence, a topic treated more fully below in the section on clinical implications.

Reaffirming

During funerals, like the rest of the grief process, great emphasis is placed not just on recounting stories but also on reaffirming values. Grief involves consideration (and reconsideration) of life's values and the spiritual moorings that provide an anchor in the loss. For many people, religious faith provides the cornerstone for this reaffirmation, and so they reaffirm their faith heritage through worship, prayer, or scripture reading. The need to find reaffirmation of beliefs and values in grief is one reason the anchor of cultural connection is so vital in the funeral experience.

Some bereaved people find reaffirmation in the inspirational writings of Helen Steiner Rice, Ralph Waldo Emerson, and John Greenleaf Whittier. The melodies and lyrics of hymns and other uplifting music also provide opportunity for reflection and reaffirmation in grief. The stirring biographies of people who overcame great odds to live out their dream and purpose for life can also be very engaging for people in grief (Smith, 2012). Even fictional superheroes can provide stirring connections for grieving individuals, both as they think through their experiences with loss and as they process their experiences with grief (Hoy, 2020; Neimeyer & Harrington, 2020).

The death of a loved one raises spiritual questions unlike any other of life's transitions. Even people who have given little thought to faith questions before find themselves grappling with those issues in bereavement. This exploration of faith is what provides the backdrop to reaffirmation, even when bereavement involves anger at God and cries about the seeming injustice of suffering.

Interestingly, during my 16 years of practice as a clinical counselor with a Southern California hospice and community bereavement organization, I found that even nonreligious people engage in this process. The fact that a bereaved parent, for example, does not have a conventional set of religious beliefs does not preclude him or her from finding spiritual meaning in the death of a child. Even though I worked with a few hundred bereaved parents in my clinical years, I do not recall a single instance in which I met a parent who, at the death of her or his child, believed that child ceased to exist. Although they might not have emotionally located that child to heaven, paradise, or a specific eternal place of bliss, every parent with whom I interacted located the dead child somewhere. Whether the child is a "star shining down at night" or a "spirit all around me," the point is that a very important spiritual exercise was being undertaken by these bereaved parents as they endeavored to make sense of their loss.

Remember that often the road to reaffirmation includes spiritual searching or even a full-blown crisis of faith. No bereavement support person should be afraid to engage bereaved people in a discussion of how they find reaffirmation in their bereavement. This making of meaning is the crux of bereavement work and often is the most complex part of the journey for bereaved individuals as they struggle to make sense of the loss and how their own life has now been so irrevocably changed by the loss (Gillies & Neimeyer, 2006).

Realizing

Because of the human tendency to deny the facts of a loved one's death, the grief process also calls the bereaved to a process of realizing the death has occurred. This is one place where the funeral with a body present (even in a closed casket) seems invaluable. Professional grief caregivers agree that, when culturally appropriate, seeing the body after death plays a vital role in this process of realization (Doka, 2002; Hoy, 2013; Hoy et al., 2021; Rando, 1984; Worden, 2018).

Even though it is helpful to see the body in a hospital bed shortly after death, my experience suggests it is also important to see the body in a casket—the most familiar symbol of death in our culture. You should be prepared for people in your work, however, for whom this experience was not possible or not chosen.

Western society is generally antagonistic to the idea of death. One poignant activity to engage in with support group participants, for example, is to invite them to share their favorite death euphemisms, the terms we use to avoid having to say that someone has died. Pointing out to those you support that our culture is not generally very comfortable with death helps explain why so many of their friends seem at a loss for words (or at least the helpful kind) or may even seem to avoid the grieving person altogether. Bereaved people will jokingly recount their favorites: *crossing over, pushing up daisies, lost him, gone to his reward,* and of course, the ubiquitous *passed away.*

Every counselor working with bereaved people has heard at least once (or maybe enumerable times) the story of bereaved people feeling the presence of their deceased loved ones. My own mother, several weeks after my dad's death, told me of her experience of hearing a car door slam outside and of going to meet him, only to realize again he had died.

Along with my brothers and me, she watched him die and she saw him in the casket at the funeral home, participating in all of those familiar rituals typical in south Louisiana. Yet, here she was, she told me, thinking at once she had surely lost her mind. It is vital to reassure bereaved individuals in our care that, like other elements of the bereavement process, the confrontation between reality and denial is an ongoing process and that these experiences do not indicate disordered grief.

Releasing

The fourth road sign indicating that grief is progressing is the growing ability to say goodbye to a loved one's physical presence and the interaction possible in human relationships. In other words, we must begin to release our loved one as we begin to move into a world from which he or she is absent. Of course, no magic formula or "do it once, get it over with" incantation exists to say goodbye.

Traditional symbols of mourning and the ceremonies of funerals help. The funeral procession, the service in a church or other familiar place, and the viewing of the body in a casket all aid in realizing that death has occurred and that the family and community relationships have been interrupted. You can also invite groups or individuals into a discussion of diverse kinds of funeral and memorial gatherings (Hoy, 2013; Long, 2009).

Saying in a support group or a training class, "Funeral and memorial ceremonies help us with our grief in many different ways. Will you tell us a little today about how your family said goodbye to your loved one?" Especially in a diverse group, the descriptions alone may elicit a lively discussion as group members hear about the customs practiced by other members of the group.

To follow up this discussion, I have often asked, "What parts of the ceremonies we have been talking about have worked for you? What parts of your own ceremonies did not seem to help? What parts of the other group members' descriptions have you particularly liked or found intriguing?" For all of their diversity, death ceremonies include some remarkably common elements in nearly all cultures. Far from being "barbaric" as some suggest, these customs provide an invaluable foundation for healing to begin.

In some ways, we spend the rest of our lives saying goodbye. Going into a restaurant frequented together requires a new widower to say goodbye. Finding "new homes" for the personal possessions treasured by her son requires a bereaved mom to say goodbye. Redecorating a room filled with reminders of the relationship shared with her husband requires a young widow to say goodbye.

The process of bereavement is really about finding new, rich ways to live life fully, even in the absence of our loved ones. This is fundamentally what release is all about.

Bereavement is fundamentally about building a bridge from the "me who used to be" to the "me who is going to be," and so, one might say, the goal of grief is fully integrating the loss into the rest of my life. Integrating is more than a goal of the grief process, but it is probably a good way to describe the "end game." The process of integrating—and really all of the process of grief—is how bereaved people live out their grief for the rest of their lives, always discovering new vistas to be enjoyed and new pathways to explore. In a word, bereaved people are not generally ruined by their losses. Instead, they are transformed by them.

Most bereaved people do exceedingly well in adjusting to their loss. The care and concern of family, friends, caregiving professionals, and volunteers, however, are of invaluable help and support as they find their way along the journey through grief.

Martyrs, Heroes, and Communal Creation of Meaning in Funerals

In a memorial obituary more than a half century after the death of Emmett Till, the *New York Times* wrote that his martyrdom, mostly viewed by the world through the images and stories emanating from his Chicago funeral, "became the rallying point for the nascent civil rights movement" (Cuba, 2016, n.p.). In spite of enumerable lynchings of Blacks at the hands of white supremacists in the early 20th century, the death of this 14-year-old boy shone a bright light on racism in America almost nine decades after African American slavery officially ended. Scholars (Holloway, 2003; Hoy, 2016; Kirk, 2013; Smith, 2010) as well as journalists (Hauck, 2020; Thomas, 1995) have long suggested that the images and stories emanating from this funeral—Till's wailing mother and the display of his disfigured body before hundreds of thousands of mourners—kindled the movement, providing action to his mother's plaintive words, of wanting the world to see what they had done to her boy. If the death of Emmett Till ignited the civil rights movement, the death of George Floyd 65 years later became the movement's 21st-century flashpoint.

On May 25, 2020, 46-year-old George Floyd, an African American resident of Minneapolis, Minnesota, was accused of trying to use counterfeit currency to make a purchase in a neighborhood store. The store clerk called police who responded to question Floyd who was sitting in a parked car nearby. Details of the interrogation are sketchy, but the outcome is clear: following a scuffle to get Floyd into the back of a patrol car, the arresting police officer put his knee on Floyd's neck for more than eight minutes. The action apparently restricted the 46-year-old's airway as he declared, "I can't breathe" and as he called out for his mother who died two years earlier. George Floyd was pronounced dead at a Minneapolis hospital shortly after arrival (Emmert et al., 2020; NBC News, 2020).

News media began its quest to fill in the backstory details on the lives of both the victim, George Floyd, and the video-recorded perpetrator, Derek Chauvin. Media accounts generally portrayed Floyd as a man with a celebrated high school athletic career who had run afoul of the law in his early adulthood, been incarcerated for drug charges and assault, and was more recently in the process of rebuilding his life as a minister and mentor to young men in his adopted hometown of Minneapolis (Fernandez & Burch, 2020; White, 2020). Chauvin was generally portrayed in the media as a white police officer with multiple citizen complaints in his file, at least two of which for excessive force had resulted in discipline (BBC News, 2020; White, 2020).

In his introduction to the funeral in Houston on June 9, NBC news anchor Lester Holt declared,

> Two weeks ago, [George] Floyd's life ended with him face down in the street, his neck pinned beneath the knee of a Minneapolis police officer now fired and charged with murder. And in those two weeks, Floyd has seen an extraordinary afterlife, if you will, as a symbol of police brutality and racial injustice, his name now a rallying cry for change.
>
> (NBC News, 2020, n.p.)

Like many such funerals, the "homegoing service" for George Floyd was characterized by significant calls for law enforcement reform, counteractions to what was described as long-standing racism, and demands for justice for the family. In his introduction of the Rev. Al Sharpton who would deliver the eulogy, Bishop James E. Dixon captured the hearts of millions:

> Because when George Floyd was gasping for breath, saying "I can't breathe," he was speaking the language of 400 years of Africans in this country. We couldn't breathe on the slave ships. We could not breathe in Jim Crow. We could not breathe through segregation. We couldn't breathe through mass incarceration.
>
> (C-SPAN, 2020, 3:24:30)

Themes of justice also often appear in these funeral ceremonies as the senseless death of the deceased issues in a call for justice, often including words such as those from the Hebrew prophet Amos who intoned, "Let justice roll down like waters, and righteousness like an ever-flowing stream" (Amos 5:24, KJV), a clear call for all people everywhere to be treated equally and fairly.

Perhaps what most characterizes the martyr funeral is a characteristic in common with funerals for military personnel and firefighters killed in the line of duty. Like their counterpart in martyr funerals, these "hero funerals" tend to personify the deceased as a larger-than-life "world changer." Funeral directors and clergy respondents recounted many experiences of a young Marine killed in combat, perhaps known to fewer than 50 family members and friends whose funeral attracts the attendance of hundreds, even if many dozens simply stand in respect on the roadside as the funeral procession passes by. In eulogies and funeral sermons at such ceremonies, these brief lives are recalled as heroes who "gave their all" in the cause of freedom or by sacrificing their lives in the rescue of others.

Near the end of his eulogy for George Floyd, Sharpton rhetorically spoke directly to the deceased when he said,

> George, I read it on the front page of the *New York Times* this morning you said you wanted to touch the world. Well, God had already made you for that. . . . George, they're marching with your name. You've touched the world in South Africa. You touched the world in England. You've touched every one of the 50 states. Even in a pandemic, people are walking out in the streets, not even following social distancing, because you've touched the world.
>
> (C-SPAN, 2020, 4:06:10)

Funerals are generally thought to be important occasions to pay tribute to the life that has been lived, and in fact, that is the source from which the contemporary notion of "celebration of life" has arisen. Whether labeling the deceased as a martyr, a hero, or some other kind of "death celebrity," honoring the character traits illustrated by specific examples from the deceased person's life seems to be what families long for in contemporary funerals. "Hearing the characteristic said aloud . . . seems to 'seal it' in the memories of the hearers more than simply mentally rehearsing the characteristics in one's own mind" (Hoy, 2013, p. 54).

How Funerals Jump-Start the Quest for Meaning

In the development and validation of their Meaning Making in Grief Scale, Yang and Lee (2022) isolated 21 items that indicate a growth in the ability of a bereaved person to create meaning in his or her loss. No fewer than the first 12 of the factors are key elements of memorial ceremonies constructed by families and communities in the immediate aftermath of death:

(1) I realized what that person meant to me; (2) I recalled good memories I had with that person which I did not know before; (3) I realized that everything I have in my life is precious; (4) I was able to recall the value of life; (5) I realized how precious that person is to me; (6) the joyful memories I had with that person became meaningful; (7) I thought about fully committing to the present moment; (8) I was able to see life with a bigger lens; (9) the grateful feelings I was not able to express toward that person came up; (10) I became more focused on the present moment than on the future; (11) I have begun to fill my moments with beautiful and happy memories; and (12) I have begun to give more importance to the memories with that person (p. 188).

Whether a bereaved family calls the gathering a celebration of life, a funeral service, a memorial gathering, or some other name, these ceremonies are marked by an honoring of the deceased's legacy through the telling of stories and the sharing of memories. Moreover, family and community affirm their own and their shared faith, philosophy, and values, usually by paying tribute to those held by the deceased, and in some cases, proclaim the injustice that brought about the person's death in the first place. Although some families appear to attempt to gloss over the fact of death by telling friends, "Wear your favorite Hawaiian shirt" or by hosting the events in "happier locations" such as parks and beaches, the very presence of the gathering forces them to acknowledge that they have gathered here and now only because someone they all love has died. And together as family and community, they begin knitting together a picture of what their future life might look like in that person's absence as they "bid farewell," whether they do that by releasing white doves, scattering cremated remains, or shoveling earth on a lowered coffin.

Clinical Implications

Provocative questions encourage the sharing of these stories. Questions that will prove to be helpful in this dialogue include "What are the times of day that hold the most vivid memories for you?" and "When and where are you when you find yourself missing your loved one the most?" Some support group leaders invite participants to bring photographs to one group meeting so the group members can all "meet" the people who have been important in the lives of the other group members. Remembering the life of a loved one begins the process of finding direction in grief.

Asking bereaved individuals how their beliefs have been shaped and reshaped by loss is also an important line of conversation for clinicians. "How has your own belief system been challenged or reaffirmed by this experience?" and for those who indicate a belief in God, "Where has God been for you in this—close at hand, some distance away, or somewhere in between?" The issues of spiritual well-being and beliefs are treated in greater detail in Chapter 3.

When bereaved individuals indicate they are struggling with the absence of the deceased, these concerns can indicate struggles at the point of realizing the loss has occurred. Vitally important, however, is that clinicians reassure bereaved individuals that sensing the deceased's presence is not an indication of pathology needing to be addressed therapeutically.

Not every experience with loss occasions pleasant memories. When a relationship was characterized by disappointments and ambivalence, possibly due to addiction or abuse, the death of that individual can create a sense of gladness and relief which, in itself, could create guilt or shame. Investigating the presence of these experiences in loss can be helpful for bereaved individuals. As one patient said weeks after the death of his abusive father, "Sometimes we don't grieve what we lost; we grieve what we never had."

Reflection and Discussion

- Do you agree with the author's assertion that funerals can jump-start the meaning-making process for families and communities? Why or why not?
- What part of the author's compass model do you find most compelling? What parts would you change or adapt? Why?
- Is there actually an element of hero or martyr in every memorial ceremony in that we tend to inflate the character of the deceased to an almost larger-than-life persona? Is this helpful or unhelpful? Why?

References

BBC News. (2020, June 8). George Floyd: What we know about the officers charged over his death. https://www.bbc.com/news/world-us-canada-52969205.

Bonanno, G.A. (2009). *The other side of sadness: What the new science of bereavement tells us about life after loss*. Basic Books.

C-SPAN. (2020, June 9). George Floyd funeral service in Houston. https://www.c-span.org/video/?472882-1/george-floyd-funeral-service-houston#.

Cuba, D. (2016, August 28). Not forgotten: Emmett Till, whose martyrdom launched the civil rights movement. *New York Times*. https://www.nytimes.com/interactive/projects/cp/obituaries/archives/emmett-till.

Doka, K.J. (2002). The role of ritual in the treatment of disenfranchised grief. In K. J. Doka (Ed.), *Disenfranchised grief: New directions, challenges and strategies for practice* (pp. 135–147). Research Press.

Emmert, M., Hertel, N.G., & Reyes, L. (2020, June 4). As Minneapolis and the nation mourns, George Floyd memorial at Cup Foods is "like a Mecca." *USA Today*. https://www.usatoday.com/story/news/nation/2020/06/04/george-floyd-memorial-cup-foods-like-mecca-mourning/3143505001/.

Fernandez, M., & Burch, A.D.S. (2020, June 18). George Floyd: From "I want to touch the world" to "I can't breathe." *New York Times*. https://www.nytimes.com/article/george-floyd-who-is.html.

Gillies, J., & Neimeyer, R.A. (2006). Loss, grief, and the search for significance: Toward a model of meaning reconstruction in bereavement. *Journal of Constructivist Psychology*, 19, 31–65. https://doi.org/10.1080/10720530500311182.

Glaser, B.G. (1998). *Doing grounded theory*. Sociology Press.

Glaser, B.G., & Strauss, A.L. (1967). *The discovery of grounded theory: Strategies for qualitative research*. Aldine.

Hauck, G. (2020, June 6). Emmett Till's lynching ignited a civil rights movement; historians say George Floyd's death could do the same. *USA Today*. https://www.usatoday.com/story/news/nation/2020/06/06/george-floyd-emmett-till-deaths-inspire-calls-change-justice/3135768001/.

Holloway, K.F.C. (2003). *Passed on: African American mourning stories*. Duke University Press.

Hoy, W.G. (1993). *Your journey through grief: A personal guide for the trip*. Premier.

Hoy, W.G. (1996). *Finding direction in your grief: Charting a course for personal growth*. GriefResources.

Hoy, W.G. (2007). *Guiding people through grief*. Compass Press.

Hoy, W.G. (2013). *Do funerals matter? The purposes and practices of death rituals in global perspective*. Routledge.

Hoy, W.G. (2016). *Bereavement groups and the role of social support: Integrating theory, research, and practice*. Routledge.

Hoy, W.G. (2016, April 17). *"Goin' up yonder": Death and meaning in African American eulogies*. Paper presented at the Association for Death Education & Counseling, Minneapolis.

Hoy, W.G. (2020). A tale of two funerals: Funeral rites, rituals, and customs across the superhero universes. In J.G. Harrington & R.A. Neimeyer (Eds.), *Superhero grief: The transformative power of loss* (pp. 87–92). Routledge.

Hoy, W.G., Becker, C.B., & Holloway, M.L. (2021). Funerals and memorial rituals. In H.L. Servaty-Seib & H.L. Chapple (Eds.), *Handbook of thanatology* (3rd ed.). Association for Death Education and Counseling.

Hsieh, H.-F., & Shannon, S.E. (2005). Three approaches to qualitative content analysis. *Qualitative Health Research*, 15(9), 1277–1288.

Kirk, K.B. (2013). Eulogy as mass mobilization narrative: Performing commemorative discourse in African American civil rights funerals. (Publication No. 3563752) [unpublished doctoral dissertation, Northwestern University]. ProQuest Dissertations and Theses Global.

Janoff-Bulman, R. (1992). *Shattered assumptions: Toward a new psychology of trauma*. Free Press.

Long, T.G. (2009). *Accompany them with singing: The Christian funeral*. Westminster John Knox Press.

McClatchey, I.S., King, S., & Domby, E. (2021). From grieving to giving: When former bereavement campers return as volunteers. *Omega: Journal of Death and Dying*, 84(1), 228–244. https://doi.org/10.1177/0030222819886734.

NBC News. (2020, June 9). Live: Funeral for George Floyd. https://www.youtube.com/watch?v=mufpOyoFrrg.

Neimeyer, R.A. (2006). *Lessons of loss* (2nd ed.). Routledge.

Neimeyer, R.A. (2019). Meaning reconstruction in bereavement: Development of a research program. *Death Studies*, 43(2), 79–91. https://doi.org/10.1080/07481187.2018.1456620.

Neimeyer, R.A. (Ed.). (2001). *Meaning reconstruction and the experience of loss*. American Psychological Association Press.

Neimeyer, R.A., & Harrington, J.G. (2020). Loss and the heroic quest for meaning. In J.G. Harrington & R.A. Neimeyer (Eds.), *Superhero grief: The transformative power of loss* (pp. 23–29). Routledge.

Park, C.L. (2005). Religion as a meaning-making framework in coping with life stress. *Journal of Social Issues*, 61(4), 707–729. https://doi.org/10.1111/j.1540-4560.2005.00428.x.

Rando, T.A. (1984). *Grief, dying, and death: Clinical interventions for caregivers*. Research Press.

Shear, M.K. (2012). Getting straight about grief. *Depression & Anxiety*, 29, 461–464. https://doi.org/10.1002/da.21963.

Smith, H.I. (2012). *Borrowed narratives: Using biographical and historical grief narratives with the bereaving*. Routledge.

Smith, S.E. (2010). *To serve the living: Funeral directors and the African American way of death*. Belknap Press.

Stroebe, M., Schut, H., & Boerner, K. (2017). Cautioning health care professionals: Bereaved persons are misguided through the stages of grief. *Omega: Journal of Death & Dying*, 74(4), 455–473. https://doi.org/10.1177/0030222817691870.

Thomas, J. (1995, September 5). Emmett's legacy. *Chicago Tribune*. https://www.chicagotribune.com/news/ct-xpm-1995-09-05-9509050005-story.html.

White, D. (2020, June 5). Did George Floyd have a criminal past and what were his previous convictions? *The Sun*. https://www.the-sun.com/news/931741/did-george-floyd-have-criminal-past/.

Worden, J.W. (2018). *Grief counseling and grief therapy: A handbook for the mental health practitioner* (5th ed.). Springer.

Wortman, J.H., & Park, C.L. (2009). Religion/spirituality and change in meaning after bereavement: Qualitative evidence for the meaning making model. *Journal of Loss & Trauma*, 14, 17–34. https://doi.org/10.1080/15325020802173876.

Yang, N.Y., & Lee, S.M. (2022). The development and validation of the Meaning Making in Grief Scale. *Death Studies*, 46(1), 178–188. https://doi.org/10.1080/07481187.2020.1725929.

Chapter 3

Memorials and the Ever-Changing Landscape of Spirituality and Faith

Arya's husband was in his upstairs study working while she was tending to household matters downstairs. It was mid-afternoon, and they planned a delightful evening out for dinner with their son and his fiancée to quietly celebrate their engagement. When Sanjay realized he had not heard from Arya in a while, he went looking, only to find she had apparently collapsed in the kitchen while she was making tea, apparently from a massive heart attack.

Even though a successful business leader and entrepreneur who had always been able to "make things happen," Sanjay was understandably shocked and devastated by the experience and overwhelmed at his sense of helplessness at seeing his wife's lifeless body. Sanjay was dazed at the death of his beloved Arya, but he knew instinctively that he could reach into the deeply held Hindu beliefs the couple shared, and he looked to the customs and rituals of a funeral to help himself, his family, his coworkers, and his friends navigate the profound loss (Arnold, 2016; Brekke, 2019; Laungani & Laungani, 2015).

Even through his shock and grief, Sanjay seemed to know intuitively that his Hindu faith would see him through his experience. With a heritage stretching back more than two millennia, the Hindu faith's sacred scriptures, beliefs, perspectives on life and death, and ceremonies provided a "compass," Sanjay would later report. Since he remembered from earlier deaths in his family that he must release his beloved Arya's spirit from her now lifeless body, he knew instinctively he must arrange for her cremation quickly, despite first responders telling him he would need to wait for the county medical examiner to complete an investigation and, likely, an autopsy.

Sanjay had a model. When his uncle had died a few years earlier in India, his family had taken advantage of the webcam service at the cremation grounds in Sidhpur, Gujarat to allow extended family living around the world to participate in the cremation rituals virtually (Scheifinger, 2019, pp. 166–168). Although he knew that an open-air cremation on a wooden pyre would likely be prohibited in the community where he

DOI: 10.4324/9781003353010-4

and Arya now lived, having been able to view the traditional rituals at least gave him a model, and he had thought much about his uncle's cremation in recent years.

The small funeral chapel was filled to overflowing as prayers were offered, sacred verses were read, and stories were shared. In keeping with their custom, Sanjay and his son wore white, as did most other family members and friends from their community who were in attendance. The family's priest led the service as mourners placed flowers inside Arya's open casket and as they laid rice balls in the casket. The priest lit a candle that was placed near Arya's head, a symbol of her life and the escape of her spirit from the body that housed it that would take place during her cremation later that morning. The assembled mourners sat cross-legged on the floor around Arya's casket. When the last prayers were offered, the funeral director and priest led the casket and mourners down a short hallway to the crematory. After the simple wooden casket was placed into the cremation chamber, Sanjay and Arya's son pushed the button that began the cremation, a Western concession to the ancient Hindu custom of a son lighting the funeral pyre for his parent (Laungani & Laungani, 2015).

In the custom of their Indian homeland, the family and community shared food and prayers throughout the next 13 days as friends from their community visited and offered support and told stories. At the end of that intense mourning period, the temple's priest led a simple prayer service in the family home, and Sanjay began the slow process of returning to work. About a month after Arya's death, Sanjay and his son took Arya's cremated remains, boarded a jetliner, and flew to Varanasi, the most sacred city along India's Ganges River. There, they offered prayers and distributed Arya's cremated remains into the flowing waters of the Ganges, following the customs of millennia—the practices their ancestors had followed for more generations than either would be able to recall (Arnold, 2016; Gawande, 2014).

As expected, Sanjay's deep Hindu spirituality meant that he regularly read and studied the sacred texts of Hinduism, the Vedas. Years after his wife's death, Sanjay still recalls both the sadness and the meaningful ceremony that were woven together in that early period of mourning in his and his family's life. His own spiritual quest has led him to write poetry about his grief and his spirituality as he learns how to continue the process discussed in chapter one of integrating his wife's death into the remaining years of his life. He talks often about how the writings of the Bhagavad Gita and other sacred texts of his faith provide solace and direction in the new life chapter he is now writing.

The deepening of Sanjay's spirituality in the aftermath of Arya's death is a common experience. Park (2005) surveyed extant clinical research and scholarly reflections on the role of religion, finding that religion had been helpful for many individuals in coping with life stresses including those who apprise faith meanings in adversity. For this population, faith helps them negotiate suffering, loss, and grief (p. 711).

Spiritual Traditions and the Value of Meaning Creation

Among professionals who care for the dying and bereaved, the terms "religion" and "spirituality" are frequently blended. For the purposes of this book and chapter, "spiritual traditions" are collectively understood to include values, beliefs, and observances that provide an individual with an ultimate sense of reality and meaning. From this vantage point, one can see why religion, spirituality, and meaning creation are so intricately linked.

Beliefs and practices include enumerable issues that are significant in caring for and supporting individuals facing death and loss. Where the dead go following physical death—if they go anywhere—is a vital question religious communities and spiritual belief systems seek to answer. Whether the afterlife is defined in terms such as "heaven," "paradise," or "a happy land," belief in the existence of such positive places or concepts make a critical difference in how a bereaved person understands a loved one's death. Nešporova (2007) posited that despite the Czech Republic's 40-year history of communism, funerals are inextricably tied to beliefs about the afterlife. Although 59% of the population claims to be non-believing, studies demonstrate that many of these "nonbelievers" actually hold varied blends of Christian (usually Catholic) beliefs, magic, occult, and Eastern religious practices.

Some traditional belief systems require prescribed rituals following death, not so much for the benefit of the bereaved family and community but to assure the safe passage of the dead to this afterlife. Bliatout (1993) noted the importance of using the correct species of tree for the Hmong decedent's coffin in order to assure that the spirit of the deceased would find the correct clan of ancestors in the afterlife. The language of ritual employed in some religious communities is crafted both to comfort bereaved family members and friends and to provide needed ministry for the deceased persons themselves.

> Having heard the word of God proclaimed and preached, the assembly responds at the vigil and at the funeral liturgy with prayers of intercession for the deceased and all the dead, for the family and all who mourn, and for all in the assembly. The holy people of God, confident in their belief in the communion of the saints, exercise their royal priesthood by joining together in this prayer for all those who have died.
>
> (Catholic Church, 1989, p. 9, § 20)

Bereavement scholars and clinicians understand the inseparability of culture and religion. Parkes and colleagues (1996, 2015) recognized how religious beliefs are woven into the fabric of death rituals, acknowledging with others that funeral rites historically have grown out of religious belief, largely due to the instinctive human need to make meaning of the unfathomable depths of death. Cultural anthropologists have long understood religious systems as social mechanisms developed to make meaning of death, even if most religious believers would object to such a humanistic defining of the history of religious faith (Pargament, 1997).

Across four decades, Pargament and colleagues have studied the effects of religious faith on coping with adverse life events. They found that positive religious coping (including forgiveness, the seeking of spiritual support, collaborating with others in coping, and benevolent religious reappraisal) was generally associated with indices of positive psychological functioning and especially of the construct of perceived post-traumatic growth (Pargament, 2022; Pargament et al., 1998). Pargament (1997, p. 3) suggested that one of religion's most salient roles in the face of crisis is using beliefs to either *conserve* or *transform* the crisis. Whereas most of these studies have been based on North American samples, more recent attempts have explored similar links between positive religious coping and positive growth after adverse events on non-Western people groups including samples from Colombia, Indonesia, South Africa, and Ukraine (Voytenko et al., 2023).

One recent study examined the influence of Bible reading on respondents' coping with difficult experiences such as deaths of friends and family members, marital separation/divorce, serious illness, and long-term unemployment. Responses from a cross-sectional study of more than 2,000 American adults indicated that frequent Bible reading was correlated with lower levels of stress after challenging life events, apparently explained, at least in part, by the religious reappraisal and the growth of personal hope that such reading seemed to produce. These results seemed to occur irrespective of the regularity of religious attendance (Krause & Pargament, 2018).

This published evidence is corroborated by interviews with funeral service professionals who indicate that bereaved families often want some spiritual leadership employed in funeral rituals, even when the deceased and often the bereaved family are not overtly religious. Funeral service professionals from rural and traditional communities across North America interviewed have reported that religiously unaffiliated families often ask for a minister for the service. In more urban and suburban North American communities, funeral homes increasingly employ the services of one or more celebrants who serve families unaffiliated with traditional faith communities but who seek a generically spiritual presider to officiate for the service.

Many celebrants see their work as highly spiritual in that they help families and communities honor the life of the deceased and find meaning in the experience of their loved one's death. Often, these celebrants are asked by families to utilize elements of more traditional religious life such as a reading of a sacred text or a poem, frequently with some reference to the sublime afterlife of the deceased. Scholarly studies at the intersection of death, spirituality, and funeral ceremonies corroborate these observations among a variety of cultural groups (Hoy, 2013; Nešporova, 2007; Okafor, 2013).

Catholicism, "Ritual Freedom," and the Role of Ceremony at Death

Less liturgical religious communities may not have a prescribed set of funeral practices expected to be in use regardless of who dies. Groups such as Evangelical and Pentecostal Christians generally celebrate the autonomy of the local congregation in such matters as visitation, funeral, and burial services As a result, their ceremonies surrounding death incorporate local customs as well as deathways that are deeply embedded in cultural and religious history. The experiences of African Americans explored more fully in Chapter 8 is a notable example of these "free church" traditions. Although there may be deep similarities from one congregation to another, each faith community's approach to funerals is distinct.

On the other hand, some faith groups have developed deeply ritualized liturgies with highly prescribed protocols to memorial rites that transcend local custom. The Roman Catholic Church is likely the best-known example of such prescribed practice, but there are similar shared rituals among Orthodox communities (Russian Orthodox, Greek Orthodox, Armenian congregations, and the like), among Anglican and Episcopal Churches, and to perhaps a lesser extent, among communities whose worship experiences are codified in a "book of order" or other such system (Lutherans, Presbyterians, and Methodists).

Although some local alteration to the prescribed liturgy may be permitted, funerals for Roman Catholic are strikingly similar around the globe, regardless of national or ethnic heritage. The approved English-language text for Roman Catholic funerals is the *Order of Christian Funerals* (Catholic Church, 1989), which both lays out the specific elements of the ritual and carefully explains the theological and historical reasons for the observances.

Traditionally among Roman Catholics, the funeral included three separate ceremonies. The vigil service, typically held the evening before the funeral mass, is a gathering for prayers, scripture reading, remembrances, and music. This ceremony often includes recitation of devotional prayers such as the rosary as well. Despite the service being called a "vigil" officially, some traditional Roman Catholics still refer to this service as "the rosary."

The second element of the Catholic ritual is the funeral mass, traditionally conducted during the morning hours. This funeral liturgy typically begins with the "reception" of the body by the parish priest at the door of the church, a ritual that is accompanied by symbolic recollection of deceased's baptism. The solemn procession of the body down the aisle of the church toward the altar is itself a reflection of the deceased's life journey of faith. During the funeral liturgy itself, scripture is read, music is shared, and prayers are offered. Typically, the eucharistic meal is shared as the gathered community celebrates the summit of Catholic worship when the bread and wine are believed to be transubstantiated—that is, actually become the body and blood of Christ. This sacred ritual is essential to many Roman Catholics' belief that their loved one reaches paradise, an eternal state of coexistence with God and all the saints.

The third element of the Roman Catholic funeral, the Rite of Committal, includes prayers and final blessings either at the grave site for earth burial or at a columbarium or crypt for cremated remains. After the three rituals are finished, many bereaved families gather in their parish hall or the family home for a meal. In practice, these three ceremonies are sometimes eclipsed into one or two. Sometimes the vigil or rosary is held in the half hour before mass begins. Sometimes the prayers of the Rite of Committal are shared before the people disperse at the end of mass, especially if the body is still to be cremated or the cemetery is located geographically distant from the church.

In Roman Catholic funeral liturgy, the morning mass is most likely to be viewed by non-Catholics as "the service" they are most likely to attend. What is conspicuous by its absence is an extended eulogy. Services in other religious communities and in nonreligious communities alike often feature one or more addresses by clergy/celebrants, family members, or friends of the deceased that essentially recount the biographical facts of the deceased's life and often extol this person's essential character qualities; see the description of the Reverend Billy Graham's funeral below for an example. In many nonliturgical funeral ceremonies, these celebratory speeches are the central feature of the gathering but not so in the Roman Catholic liturgy.

In fact, *Order of Christian Funerals* expressly forbids the inclusion of a eulogy during the funeral liturgy, choosing instead for the homilist (celebrant) to focus on God's compassionate love, the message of the gospel, and Jesus's victory over death through resurrection (Catholic Church, 1989, p. 8, § 27). The prescribed liturgy does permit an inclusion of remembrances by family or friends, typically near the end of the funeral liturgy after communion is received by the entire community in attendance (Catholic Church, 1989, p. 89, § 170). Although Roman Catholic liturgy does not include eulogy per se, priests who know the deceased personally often weave significant elements from the deceased's character and behavior into the homily in just the same ways other ministers, rabbis, and celebrants weave these elements into their own addresses.

Some Protestant ministers and Jewish rabbis purposefully weave characteristics honored in the faith (generosity, faithfulness, integrity) with stories and anecdotes from the deceased's life to create a picture of the deceased in the context of faith. Long (2009) decried any focus on pastimes and hobbies in the funeral, declaring that the Christian funeral should emphasize the life of faith. Some recount choosing a specific person in sacred scripture and relating that story to the deceased during the funeral ceremony (Hoy, 2008; Lloyd, 1997).

Order of Christian Funerals goes to great length to explain the theological significance of the symbols and liturgical movements of the funeral. Symbols such as a funeral pall (when local custom utilizes it), the printed Book of the Gospels, holy water, incense, and the paschal candle are briefly explained. Depending on the presider's sense of the number of non-Catholics in attendance, the significance of these symbols are often explained to the gathered mourners as well. As an example, the *Order of Christian Funerals* explains the use of incense as a symbol of honor to the deceased body and as a symbolic reminder of the people's prayers ascending to God (Catholic Church, 1989, p. 10, § 37).

The Roman Catholic Church also states its clear "preference" about how deceased bodies are cared for and their final disposition. Because the human was "marked" with the seal of the Trinity in baptism and became the temple of the Holy Spirit, the Church explains, customs related to how the body is prepared must be marked with respect and honor. Although the Church permits cremation (except when chosen for "anti-Christian motives"), the Church clearly prefers that historical Christian precedent be followed by burying or entombing the body (Catholic Church, 1989, p. 6, § 19).

In response to a growing practice of cremation among Catholics in the United States, Canada, the United Kingdom, Australia, and New Zealand, the Church published its *Cremation Appendix* several years after the revised funeral liturgy was published. This document clearly noted that although cremation is permitted, the practice "does not enjoy the same value as burial of the body" (Catholic Church, 1997, § 413). In their subsequent explanation of the Church's official tenets by the U.S. Conference of Catholic Bishops (2023), the bishops soundly rejected the scattering of cremated remains, the retention at home or any other non-sacred space of cremated remains, or the division of cremated remains among family members—for example, in "keepsake urns." In a clear rebuke to what Church leaders had apparently heard in the personal theologies of some Catholics, they explained, "The body is not something that is used temporarily by the soul as a tool and that can ultimately be discarded as no longer useful" (p. 1).

Citing its belief in the sacredness of the body and the importance of the remains—cremated or buried whole—staying intact (insofar as death circumstances permit), the 2023 clarification further prohibited American Catholics in practicing alkaline hydrolysis and human composting because they fail to provide adequate witness to the belief in resurrection (p. 4). The guidelines go on to explain that one problematic feature in these dispositions, shared with the practice of "scattering" cremated remains, is that there is no "sacred place" where mourners can visit for prayer and remembrance (p. 5).

Like with members of other religious systems, adherents to Roman Catholicism represent a wide range of opinions on how closely to follow the bishops' instructions. As one priest commented, "The distance from pulpit to pew is often about 1,000 miles." Older, more traditionally minded Catholics are likely more inclined to follow the Church's edicts without question. Likewise, funeral professional and clergy respondents note that recent immigrants tend to select more traditional funeral options, even though these populations may struggle financially more than established bereaved families, a topic explored in more detail in Chapter 5.

Although sometimes criticized as "impersonal" by those who are unfamiliar with highly prescribed rituals such as those practiced by the Roman Catholic or Orthodox Churches, there are clear benefits to such order. The period of early bereavement is filled with chaos for bereaved families and communities, and this chaos is exacerbated when the death is unexpected. Even months and years after the death, one common sentiment expressed in interviews with bereaved members of these faith communities is the sense of calm and order offered by the predictability of the ritual. One funeral director expressed, "It is as if the Church is standing in the center aisle [showing his arms outstretched] saying, 'As a community of faith, we have been here before. Follow us as we show you the way through.'"

One of the reasons these highly prescribed rituals likely offer calm is due to the reduced choices that must be made in early bereavement. Whether the death was expected, there are extensive lists across the internet of the 50 or 100 decisions that must be made in the first 48 hours after a death. Although some of these choices are not alleviated by prescribed rituals, many of them (place of rites, scripture to be read, order of service, and music selections) are either eliminated by the prescribed ritual or at least reduced to a manageable few. The Roman Catholic funeral liturgy, for example, offers a selection of appropriate biblical readings to be used during the funeral liturgy from which the family can choose, greatly reducing the chaos of having to scramble in the family Bible to "find Mom's favorites."

While results are mixed, many studies indicate that acute stress complicates decision making. Some studies have demonstrated that high levels of stress cause individuals to make riskier decisions than they would otherwise or to experience a near paralysis of decision-making ability (Porcelli & Delgado, 2017).

Highly prescribed rituals also offer members of the larger community a ready framework for providing support. Anecdotally, some individuals have reported they are more likely to attend a funeral when "I know what will happen," reflecting a general human tendency to prefer the "known to the unknown." This phenomenon also might be a concession to individuals with highly scheduled lives who reward with their attention those events that have a prescribed beginning and ending. If a memorial gathering's attendance is increased based on these expectations, the sense of social support experienced by bereaved family members is generally enhanced. One father reported how moved he was as they followed his son's casket into the church and realized the church was full (Hoy, 2013).

Ceremonies in Christian Free Protestant Traditions

Unlike Roman Catholic funerals, Christian Protestant funerals—especially those in the so-called free church tradition such as Evangelical and Pentecostal congregations—are typically free from the ritual formality of a prescribed liturgy. Rather than using formal guidelines from the global church, local clergy and family collaborate on the elements of the service and the specific order for their inclusion. Although the various branches of Christian faith share common elements of the memorial ceremony—prayers, scripture reading, music, and one or more funeral "orations" in the form of homily, sermon, funeral message, and eulogy—the composition of these and the order in which they are placed can be highly varied.

Despite their lack of ritual order, however, Protestant funeral ceremonies in the free church tradition tend to follow a typical organization with music, scripture, and prayers interspersed through the first portion of the service followed by a funeral sermon or eulogy. In most observed free Protestant congregations or ceremonies, this funeral sermon, usually lasting between 10 and 20 minutes, is based on a passage of sacred scripture the minister reads and often then relates to the deceased's life. Sometimes parallels are drawn between a biographical scripture passage (such as the Hebrew faith characters Joseph, Moses, David, or Ruth) and the deceased person.

In one such example, the pastor read a short portion of scripture from the Bible: "And [God] raised up David to be their king, of whom he testified and said, 'I have found in David the son of Jesse a man after my heart, who will do all my will'" (Acts 13:22, ESV). The pastor explained the context of the verse as a sermon from Paul the apostle and then went on to explain why the Bible calls David a "man after God's own heart." The pastor acknowledged David was an imperfect man but explained three characteristics the pastor observed in David's life that could be imitated in mourners' lives: his trust in God, his faithfulness, and his desire for worship. With each characteristic from David's life, the pastor pointed to an example of that characteristic from the deceased man's life and encouraged the congregation to imitate that character.

When world-famous Evangelical preacher Billy Graham died at age 99 in 2018, more than 2,000 family members, friends, and invited guests gathered under a giant canopy to pay tribute. The enormous tent was reminiscent of the tent under which Graham preached his first "crusades" in the late 1940s before moving to large stadiums. The funeral was held on the grounds of the Billy Graham Library in North Carolina in front of the Graham family home which had been moved and reassembled. The centerpiece of the funeral was the pulpit from which Billy Graham preached in the latter part of his ministry standing just behind Graham's simple casket, made by inmates at Louisiana's Angola State Penitentiary.

A decade before his death, Graham had worked with other family members to plan the funeral, determining with them who would speak and what music would be shared. In keeping with these plans, each of his five children spoke, though his eldest son and namesake, Franklin Graham, delivered the main funeral sermon.

Like his father before him, Franklin Graham shared a simple, declarative message of belief in the Bible, of the power of sin in people's lives, and of the only remedy to that sin being repentance and faith in Jesus Christ. "The world, with all of its political correctness, would want you to believe that there are many roads to God. It's just not true," Graham declared (Foreman & Drew, 2018, n.p.). Throughout Graham's sermon and the testimonies of the other children, the attendees and the world was assured "there were not two Billy Grahams"—the Billy Graham that the world saw on the big stage was the same Billy Graham his family saw at home.

Music included simple piano arrangements of Christian hymns and gospel songs, as well as vocalists such as the Gaither Vocal Band of male singers, who intoned the gospel song "The Love of God." Prayers and reflections were offered by ministers who were friends and colleagues in ministry. Following the final prayer of benediction, the strains of "Amazing Grace" played by a lone bagpiper led casket and family away from the tent to the grave site in the woods next to Graham's wife, Ruth, who died eleven years earlier (Foreman & Drew, 2018; Gjelten, 2018).

Spiritual Challenges in Memorial Ceremonies

Some results suggest participation in meaningful funeral ceremonies improves clinical outcomes for bereaved people (Fristad et al., 2001; Gamino et al., 2000; Hoy, 2013). In their study of Catholic bereaved families and mortuary workers in Cebu, Philippines during the COVID-19 pandemic, Boholano and Bacus (2022) found that health restrictions significantly limited traditional practices among these highly family-oriented Catholic mourners. Long wakes, hospitality of the bereaved family toward their sympathizers, and other traditional rites of mourning were significantly compromised because of health restrictions, with the authors concluding, "The deprivation of performing the rituals and public gatherings of grief was regarded as unfinished mourning. With the loss, the bereaved family did not enjoy the presence of others. They were left alone to cope with their grief" (pp. 10623–10624). The experience of these Filipino Catholic families was repeated hundreds of thousands of times with other bereaved families during this period, a phenomenon addressed fully in Chapter 7.

Potential challenges arise in the bereavement outcomes among individuals whose beliefs and practices do not follow the majority family opinion. Some bereaved individuals have experienced their grief as the outliers because most other family members have held a religious belief dramatically different than theirs. Sometimes, these individuals have disaffiliated with all faith communities finding none to be satisfactory; other times, these individuals have left the faith of their family of origin, and as a result, the death rituals of that more traditional religious community no longer meet their needs.

For example, one woman had become an Evangelical Protestant after attending a Billy Graham Evangelistic Crusade. She described how unsatisfactory she had found the traditional rituals of her mother's Roman Catholic Church. Ironically, she noted, even her nominally active siblings seemingly derived little meaning from the funeral.

What became clear during her discussions with a grief counselor was that the bereaved daughter was not just dissatisfied with the "impersonal" nature of the prescribed funeral liturgy. She also had significant reservations about her deceased mother's faith and whether her mother was eternally "saved" since in the daughter's new tradition, a personal conversion experience was necessary. The daughter was sure that her mother had never identified having had such an experience, and her lack of confidence about her mother's eternal destiny complicated her experience with grief even beyond her dissatisfaction with the funeral.

The "nominally Catholic" bereaved siblings the daughter identified were, according to her, not satisfied with the rigidity of the funeral liturgy either. At the funeral mass, her brother wanted to project the video he had created with a photo montage set to the music of some of her mother's favorite show tunes. He was told that was not possible. Although the funeral director did arrange to show the video at the vigil service and visitation the night before, many of the deceased's older friends did not attend because the service was after dark, essentially leaving them out of the part of the funeral that some in the family found most meaningful, according to the family report.

Sometimes, funeral directors reach out to leadership of large congregations because the death of a young person or an unusually notable community member will occasion a large funeral gathering. When the deceased and family do not have a congregation of their own, these funeral directors look to these large congregations, which are usually Evangelical Christian churches because their large worship centers often will accommodate hundreds of mourners.

Some of these faith community leaders, however, find these requests difficult to fulfill. In an interview, one pastor expressed it this way: "It is true we have a large building, but our church is not just a venue for gatherings. It is a sacred space that is dedicated to expressing our faith in a Christ-honoring way. I have to be very careful about what message is proclaimed from that pulpit because that will be seen by the people attending as a message our church believes."

Funeral directors and clergy need to work together serving bereaved families rather than at cross-purposes. Some funeral directors partner with clergy to communicate why services held within the sacred house of worship should employ music, readings, and speakers affirming the deceased person's faith. Songs such as Roy Rogers and Dale Evans's "Happy Trails to You" played at the end of a funeral might neither be an affirmation of the congregation's faith nor the pastor's personal preference, but allowing this music might actually mitigate bereavement distress.

Clinical Implications

Dissatisfaction with the funeral and other adverse events related to the intersection of religious faith and memorial ceremonies are important topics of consideration for clinicians. Clinicians are wise to ask early in the assessment interview with a newly bereaved individual, "Would you tell me about the funeral or memorial ceremony?" and then follow that response with "In what ways did you find the ceremony helpful to you, and what would you have changed if you could?" The responses to these questions will often reveal both the elements of funeral ceremonies the bereaved individual has perceived as supportively helpful and the parts that they might classify as an "adverse event" (Gamino et al., 2000).

Vieten and colleagues (2016) found that matters of religious faith are addressed by only a slim minority of practicing clinical psychologists despite the religiosity of patients and the desire of most patients to address these matters in their counseling. Oxhandler and Parrish (2018) found that a significant minority of psychologists, licensed clinical social workers, licensed professional counselors, licensed marriage and family counselors, and advanced practice nurses utilized spirituality in any significant ways in their practices. Fewer than half of social workers and licensed marriage and family therapists self-reported conducting a full psycho-social-spiritual assessment on every client and only about one-third of psychologists and licensed professional counselors reported that they did (p. 689).

Because data show that the majority of patients/clients want their spiritual issues sensitively addressed in their care, clinicians must find ways to incorporate spiritual assessments into their intake and counseling processes (Balboni et al., 2017; Sulmasy, 2002). One tool that is widely available for use to clinicians is the F.I.C.A. spiritual assessment framework developed by Pulchalski (2006) and tested in subsequent studies (Borneman et al., 2010). The simple pattern of F.I.C.A. inquires whether the patient endorses faith or beliefs (F), asks about the importance of those beliefs and practices (I), discovers if there is a faith community or faith leader with whom the patient identifies a connection (C), and queries how the patient wants these issues addressed in care (A) (Pulchalski, 2006, p. 153).

All counselors who support bereaved individuals are well advised to inquire as to the importance and role employed by spiritual meaning in the individual's life and experience. Inquiring about which sacred scriptures or music have proven helpful can provide an important discussion point about the role of spiritual beliefs in the bereaved person's life. Many bereaved individuals describe their use of the Psalms, the poetry shared by Jews and Christians alike, in their own devotional reading, and many books have been published that analyze the 40 or so psalms of lament (Brueggemann, 1984; Card, 2005; Jinkins, 1998; Westermann, 1981).

For bereaved individuals who found the religious components of the ceremony to be less than satisfactory, as well as for those who did not have a service, clinicians will want to continually build skills in helping their clients and patients develop personally meaningful therapeutic rituals. When the above counseling question ending with "what would you change if you could?" is answered with specific ideas, clinicians can join the bereaved individual in cocreating a meaningful ritual to be used in therapy. This ritual might include texts, music played from a mobile device playlist, and even a eulogy written for the deceased and read aloud in the counseling room.

One of the greatest temptations facing care providers is the assumption that in understanding a few basics about a cultural or religious group, one understands the bereavement experiences of those individuals who practice that cultural custom. The voluminous literature on cultural awareness has shifted from early assumptions that cultural competence was achievable to a more realistic understanding that the best one can hope for is cultural humility (Green-Moton & Minkler, 2020). In an attempt to become "culturally competent," professionals must avoid the trap of "trading in one set of stereotypes for another" (Hoy, 2013, p. 3).

One recent effort to create balance in this conundrum is what Hoy et al. (2024, in process) call "cultural attunement" wherein clinicians work to be humble in their outlook—"I do not really know your culture because my vision is clouded by my own background"—and culturally curious by asking sensitive questions as a learner seeking to be instructed by the client.

Reflection and Discussion

- What are the spiritual beliefs you hold that are most important in facing death and loss? How have you seen these change over your lifetime?
- When has been a time in your life that your spiritual beliefs were significantly challenged by something that happened in your personal life, your family, your community, or the world? How did you work through this "crisis of belief"?
- Which spiritual beliefs related to death and loss do you find most difficult to understand or support?
- How would the notions of cultural humility and/or cultural attunement inform care of the bereaved that are sensitive to the individual's spiritual beliefs? How does this potentially prevent crossing boundaries in the counselor's relationship with the bereaved person?

References

Arnold, D. (2016). Burning issues: Cremation and incineration in modern India. *Naturwissenschaften, Technik und Medizin*, 24(4), 393–419. https://doi.org/10.1007/s00048-017-0158-7.

Balboni, T.A., Fitchett, G., Handzo, G.F., Johnson, K.S., Koenig, H.G., Pargament, K. I., Puchalski, C.M., Sinclair, S., Taylor, E.J., & Steinhauser, K.E. (2017). State of the science of spirituality and palliative care research part II: Screening, assessment, and interventions. *Journal of Pain and Symptom Management*, 54(3), 441–453. https://doi.org/10.1016/j.jpainsymman.2017.07.029.

Bliatout, B.T. (1993). Hmong death customs: Traditional and acculturated. In D.P. Irish, K.F. Lundquist, & V.J. Nelsen (Eds.), *Ethnic variations in dying, death, and grief: Diversity in universality* (pp. 79–100). Taylor & Francis.

Boholano, H.B., & Bacus, R.C. (2022). Catholic funeral traditions and alterations due to the COVID-19 pandemic: Implications to compliance to health protocols. *Journal of Positive School Psychology*, 6(6), 10614–10630. https://journalppw.com/index.php/jpsp/article/view/9688.

Borneman, T., Ferrell, B., & Pulchalski, C.M. (2010). Evaluation of the FICA tool for spiritual assessment. *Journal of Pain & Symptom Management*, 40(2), 163–173. https://doi.org/10.1016/j.jpainsymman.2009.12.019.

Brekke, T. (2019). *The Oxford history of Hinduism: Modern Hinduism*. Oxford University Press. https://doi.org/10.1093/oso/9780198790839.001.0001.

Brueggemann, W. (1984). *The message of the Psalms: A theological commentary*. Augsburg.

Card, M. (2005). *A sacred sorrow: Reaching out to God in the lost language of lament*. NavPress.

Catholic Church. (1989). *Order of Christian funerals: Study edition*. Liturgy Training Publications.

Catholic Church. (1997). *Order of Christian funerals: Appendix—cremation*. Liturgy Training Publications.

Foreman, T., & Drew, J. (2018, March 2). Watch: The Rev. Billy Graham's funeral. *PBS News Hour*. https://www.pbs.org/newshour/nation/watch-live-the-rev-billy-grahams-funeral.

Fristad, Cerel, J., Goldman, M., Weller, E.B., & Weller, R.A. (2001). The role of ritual in children's bereavement. *Omega: Journal of Death and Dying*, 42(4), 321–339. https://doi.org/10.2190/MC87-GQMC-VCDV-UL3U.

Gamino, L.A., Easterling, L.W., Stirman, L.S., & Sewell, K.W. (2000). Grief adjustment as influenced by funeral participation and occurrence of adverse funeral events. *Omega: Journal of Death and Dying*, 41(2), 79–92.

Gawande, A. (2014). *Being mortal: Medicine and what matters in the end*. Henry Holt.

Gjelten, T. (2018, March 2). Billy Graham's funeral celebrated evangelist's life and the reach of his ministry. *NPR All Things Considered*. https://www.npr.org.

Green-Moton, E., & Minkler, M. (2020). Cultural competence or cultural humility? Moving beyond the debate. *Health Promotion Practice*, 21(1), 142–145. https://doi.org/10.1177/1524839919884912.

Hoy, W.G. (2008). *Road to Emmaus: Pastoral care with the dying and bereaved*. Compass Press.

Hoy, W.G. (2013). *Do funerals matter? The purposes and practices of death rituals in global perspective*. Routledge.

Hoy, W.G., Clemons, M.K., & Gamino, L.A. (2024, in process). A call for cultural attunement for thanatologists.

Jinkins, M. (1998). *In the house of the Lord: Inhabiting the Psalms of lament*. Liturgical Press.

Krause, N., & Pargament, K.I. (2018). Reading the Bible, stressful life events, and hope: Assessing an overlooked coping resource. *Journal of Religion and Health*, 57(4), 1428–1439. https://doi.org/10.1007/s10943-018-0610-6.

Laungani, P., & Laungani, A. (2015). Death in a Hindu family. In C.M. Parkes, P. Laungani, & B. Young (Eds.), *Death and bereavement across cultures* (2nd ed.; pp. 42–60). Routledge.

Lloyd, D.S. (1997). *Leading today's funerals: A pastoral guide for improving bereavement ministry*. Baker.

Long, T.G. (2009). *Accompany them with singing: The Christian funeral*. Westminster John Knox Press.

Mitima-Verloop, H.B., Mooren, T.T., & Boelen, P.A. (2021). Facilitating grief: An exploration of the function of funerals and rituals in relation to grief reactions. *Death Studies*, 45(9), 735–745. https://doi.org/10.1080/07481187.2019.1686090.

Nešporova, O. (2007). Believer perspectives on death and funeral practices in a non-believing country. *Sociologický Časopis*, 43(6), 1175–1193. https://doi.org/10.13060/00380288.2007.43.6.04.

Okafor, H.C. (2013). *Perceptions of loss and grief experiences within religious burial and funeral* (Publication No. 1657) [unpublished doctoral dissertation], University of New Orleans. https://scholarworks.uno.edu/td/1657.

Oxhandler, H.K., & Parrish, D.E. (2018). Integrating clients' religion/spirituality in clinical practice: A comparison among social workers, psychologists, counselors, marriage and family therapists, and nurses. *Journal of Clinical Psychology, 74*(4), 680–694. https://doi.org/10.1002/jclp.22539.

Pargament. K.I. (1997). *The psychology of religion and coping: Theory, research, practice*. Guilford.

Pargament, K.I. (2022). The privilege of teaching: Some lessons learned from over 40 years mentoring graduate students in the clinical psychology of religion and spirituality. *Spirituality in Clinical Practice*, 9(1), 55–59. https://doi.org/10.1037/scp0000262.

Pargament, K.I., Smith, B.W., Koenig, H.G., & Perez, L. (1998). Patterns of positive and negative religious coping with major life stressors. *Journal for the Scientific Study of Religion*, 37(4), 710–724. https://doi.org/10.2307/1388152.

Park, C.L. (2005). Religion as a meaning-making framework in coping with life stress. *Journal of Social Issues*, 61(4), 707–729.

Parkes, C.M., Laungani, P., & Young, B. (Eds.). (1996). *Death and bereavement across cultures*. Routledge.

Parkes, C.M., Laungani, P., & Young, B. (Eds.). (2015). *Death and bereavement across cultures* (2nd ed.). Routledge.

Porcelli, A.J., & Delgado, M.R. (2017). Stress and decision making: Effects on valuation, learning, and risk-taking. *Current Opinion in Behavioral Sciences*, 14, 33–39. https://doi.org/10.1016/j.cobeha.2016.11.015.

Puchalski, C.M. (2001). The role of spirituality in health care. *Proceedings—Baylor University Medical Center*, 14(4), 352–357. https://doi.org/10.1080/08998280.2001.11927788.

Pulchalski, C.M. (2006). Spiritual assessment in clinical practice. *Psychiatric Annals*, 36(3), 150–155.

Scheifinger, H. (2019). Online Hinduism. In T. Brekke (Ed.), *The Oxford history of Hinduism: Modern Hinduism*. Oxford University Press. https://doi.org/10.1093/oso/9780198790839.001.0001.

Sulmasy, D.P. (2002). A biopsychosocial-spiritual model for the care of patients at the end of life. *Gerontologist*, 42(Special Issue 3), 24–33. https://doi.org/10.1093/geront/42.suppl_3.24.

U.S. Conference of Catholic Bishops, Committee on Doctrine. (2023, March 20). On the proper disposition of bodily remains. https://www.usccb.org/resources/On%20Proper%20Disposition%202023-03-20.pdf.

Vieten, C., Scammell, S., Pierce, A., Pilato, R., Ammondson, I., Pargament, K.I., & Lukoff, D. (2016). Competencies for psychologists in the domains of religion and spirituality. *Spirituality in Clinical Practice*, 3(2), 92–114. https://doi.org/10.1037/scp0000078.

Voytenko, V.L., Pargament, K.I., Cowden, R.G., Lemke, A.W., Kurniati, N.M.T., Bechara, A.O., Joynt, S., Tymchenko, S., Khalanskyi, V.V., Shtanko, L., Kocum, M., Korzhov, H., Mathur, M.B., Ho, M.Y., VanderWeele, T.J., & Worthington, E. L. (2023). Religious coping with interpersonal hurts: Psychosocial correlates of the brief RCOPE in four non-western countries. *Psychology of Religion and Spirituality*, 15(1), 43–55. https://doi.org/10.1037/rel0000441.

Westermann, C. (1981). *Praise and lament in the Psalms*. John Knox Press.

Chapter 4

Children, Teens, and Memorial Ceremonies

When a family in Chris's congregation experienced the death of a four-month-old son by sudden infant death syndrome, the young minister grappled with how to best incorporate the five older, surviving children, aged 4–12 into the funeral. The pastor remarked to the funeral director in the phone call confirming the time for the service, "I guess I was absent the day we talked about *this* in seminary." After careful consideration and conversations with the parents, Chris decided to bring the children to the front of the funeral chapel just before the funeral sermon to sing, while the congregation's pianist played the hymn "Jesus Loves Me." The favorite childhood hymn simply declares in its chorus, "Yes, Jesus loves me! Yes, Jesus loves me! / Yes, Jesus loves me! The Bible tells me so" (Warner, 1859). The little choir of voices shared comfort with gathered mourners as they expressed their own collective grief at the death of their baby brother. Perhaps the greatest gift of all, at least to the children's specialist from the local bereavement center, was that the children were not ignored in the funeral but rather were deeply engaged in its execution.

Like Chris, the young minister whose experience began this chapter, most professionals seem to have "been absent" on the day that child death was discussed in training and that leaves any caregiving professional grappling for instructions on how best to provide support. This chapter addresses the deaths of young people who die in their childhood or teen years, the bereavement experiences that are likely to be part of the family and community's journey to grapple with the loss, and the ceremonies that help these grieving persons begin to create meaning in the midst of such an unspeakable loss. This chapter also addresses what needs to be done in memorial ceremonies for children and teens who face the deaths of family members, classmates, and friends. Grieving children have been called the forgotten mourners, and my experience working with school officials, families, and faith communities indicates we are not much better at meeting the needs of teen mourners.

DOI: 10.4324/9781003353010-5

Bereavement after a Child's or Teen's Death

So infrequently do families in high-income communities experience the death of a young person that for many people, that death seems "out of order." The outcry about how wrong such a death is confirms the bias that individuals who populate these high-income communities seem to have been duped into believing the myth "Children do not die." In the United States, higher family income has been significantly associated with a lower prevalence of serious physical and mental illness as well as lower ten-year mortality rates (Udalova et al., 2022).

Residents in lower-income communities are far less likely to believe the myth that children do not die. They have attended enough funerals for children and teens that they know the bitter reality of pediatric mortality. Lower family socioeconomic status (SES) has long been noted to increase the health risks for all family members, especially children. Although in their study Braudt and colleagues (2019) conceded financial well-being was not the only predictor of high child mortality, in this survey of 377,252 children and youth aged 1–17 in the United States, young people in families living at or below the federally defined poverty level were significantly more likely to die from all causes than their high-income neighbors. In their discussion, the authors noted that their results clearly showed that when compared with higher SES peers, children living with parents with lower levels of education, in low-income households, and/or in households without two present parents "are more likely to die in early life" (Braudt et al., 2019, p. 1387).

Remes and colleagues (2011) reached similar conclusions about youth and families in Finland, finding from 15 years of data that the highest concentration of excess mortality among children was among children aged one to four living with single parents who were less educated and earned less money.

In 2021, the estimated global mortality rate for children under age five was 4 deaths per 1,000 live births in Europe, Australia, and New Zealand and 6 deaths per 1,000 births in North America. However, the under-five mortality rate was more than tenfold higher in sub-Saharan Africa at 74 deaths per 1,000 live births and in low-income countries overall at 67 deaths per 1,000 live births (UNICEF, 2023). These data are corroborated by my fieldwork in Kenya where most older mothers have had at least one child die during the mothers' lifetime. This does not make pediatric death less sad in low-income countries; it only makes it more real.

Whereas in high-income communities youth deaths are primarily from external causes (accidents, suicide, and homicides), in low-income countries, deaths of children and teens tend to far more frequently result from substandard prenatal and neonatal care, inadequate nutrition, contaminated water, and lack of medical care. Children living in what the

United Nations defines as fragile and conflict-affected situations are three times more likely to die before age five (UNICEF, 2023).

Complex Issues of Bereavement after Child Death

With youth deaths, several factors seem to make bereavement more complicated for survivors. When the death was by violent means, parents and other primary caregivers struggle to make sense of the loss and are at a higher risk of complicated grief than when the death was by natural causes (Keesee et al., 2008). In their study of 575 parents following the death of a child, Feigelman and colleagues (2011) found grief experiences are complicated, especially long lived, and marked by stigma when a child dies by suicide or substance overdose compared to those whose deaths were by accident or natural causes.

In one longitudinal study of bereaved parents, researchers found negative effects endure for the lifetime of the parents following a child's death, leading these parents to report lower overall health-related quality of life in older age than did their nonbereaved counterparts, even decades after a child's death (Song et al., 2010).

In Ho and Brotherson's (2007) interviews with ten mostly Buddhist (80%) Macau Chinese bereaved parents, two primary themes emerged in the research. First, parents sought a means to maintain a "continuing bond" (Klass et al., 1996) with the dead child, and parents sought this continuing bond through the use of linking objects (specifically photos and gifts given by the child to the parent). These linking objects were frequently shown to the interviewers by the parent. Second, parents sought ways to memorialize their child through activities and items not previously connected to the child. One mother wrote articles about her child and her feelings about the death while another purchased a memorial tablet in the local Buddhist temple in her daughter's memory.

One bereaved parent placed the urn with the child's cremated remains on a lower shelf of the family altar in the home, reserving the upper shelves for older ancestors who had previously died. The remains being situated in the family altar with older kin meant that the deceased child had incense burned daily in his honor and remembrance of him became part of the family memory (Ho & Brotherson, 2007, p. 12).

Parents are at an elevated risk of complicated grief and prolonged grief disorder following a child's death. In a cross-sectional study of bereaved individuals, Thielman and colleagues (2023) found that functional impairment as a result of parental grief was endorsed by 44.7%, although like the other symptoms of complicated grief, the levels of reported impairment tended to decline the further one got from the loss.

Complicated bereavement is not confined to parents in the aftermath of a child's death. Grandparents often report a "double loss," once for the death of their grandchild and another at witnessing the pain of their own child, the deceased child's parent (Reed, 1999). Gilrane-McGarry and O'Grady (2012, pp. 173–174) found with their sample of 17 Irish grandparents that the sense of double pain identified by Reed and others was better described as "cumulative pain" encompassing pain from five elements: previous bereavements, actual loss of the grandchild, witnessing the son's or daughter's grief, witnessing subsequent negative changing in the son or daughter, and pain that is common in all grief expressed with words like "devastation," "anger," and "resentment."

Grandparents expressed significant experiences of pain at shattered dreams accompanied by the grandchild's death. Although shattered dreams are typically considered in parental bereavement, clinicians are apt to forget these can be an important component of grandparent grief as well. Moreover, because older adults have typically experienced many losses over their lives, Gilrane-McGarry and O'Grady (2012) surmised that their research respondents brought all of those experiences to bear on the deaths of their grandchildren.

Just as grandparent grief is an understudied phenomenon, so are the bereavement experiences of siblings. The sibling relationship has been called the "most complicated of all family ties" with siblings being both friends and enemies. In their formulation of a theory about sibling bereavement in adolescence, Hogan and DeSantis (1996, p. 236) noted that in light of the size of American families, the majority of teens whose sibling dies become an only child, a trend that has intensified with smaller average family size in the 21st century. They wrote that the death of a sibling "shatters" all hope for "a shared future that is not to be" (p. 250). Even adolescent siblings can express concern about who will now help shoulder the responsibilities of caring for aging parents and carrying on the family legacy when the sibling set is reduced by a death.

The rivalry that characterized childhood, adolescence, and young adulthood is resolved by middle age for many siblings. However, when a young person's siblings die prior to this resolution, there can be significant regret and guilt in the youthful griever, who has had still-unresolved conflict with the now-deceased brother or sister. This rivalry can be especially significant when a younger sibling senses he or she "is not enough," perhaps because of "living in the shadow of comparison" to the now-deceased child's academic or athletic accomplishments (Davies, 1999; Marshall & Davies, 2011).

Bereaved children and teens frequently exhibit significant need for attention after the death of a sibling, which may be evidenced by increased aggression. Because the family system is so substantially altered by the death of a child, parents and other caregivers likely exhibit a reduced level of emotional energy to invest in relationships with surviving siblings (McCown & Davies, 1995). Interestingly, sibling behavior problems seem to be less pronounced among children and teens who were included in funeral and memorial activities versus those who were excluded (Davies, 1988, 1999).

Community Response to Pediatric Deaths

Families are widely regarded as "primary mourners," causing many observers to assume the community's role is to provide care, social support, and condolence (Zunin & Zunin, 1992). Believing the community's role is to provide support, however, may overlook the deep grief experienced by classmates, friends, and their families.

Multiple times over my career, I have been asked to address groups of parents about how to best support their own children after a classmate or friend dies, and without exception, these presentations have been made before crowded rooms. After four young people were killed in a car crash in California, I addressed almost 300 parents gathered in the school auditorium, responding to questions about appropriate behaviors and concerns parents voiced over their own adolescent children's responses to the loss. Neither these parents nor most of their children required the intervention of our clinical team. Rather, they needed another understanding parent who could utilize clinical training and experience to normalize the experiences of grief and point out "danger signs" to which they should be alert in their children. In retrospect, I suspect the greatest gift in the gatherings was the solidarity these parents gained with their own parental peers, many of whom they did not previously know.

Margola and colleagues (2010) compared written reflections from three time intervals following the classroom death of a 15-year-old boy in Italy, whose death was apparently from a substance overdose, in the presence of classmates. Seventy-seven percent of parents gave permission for their adolescent children to participate in the follow-up study, allowing the researchers to compare the reflections written by 7 male and 13 female students. Students completed reflective writing assignments on three consecutive days, approximately two weeks after the student's death. At 14 days, 24 days, and 5 months post-loss, the students also completed a self-report measure using an Italian translation of the Impact of Events Scale (Weiss & Marmar, 1997).

Analysis of the writing assignment revealed students progressed over the three days from a primarily factual account of the experience on the first day to significantly more emotional processing of the traumatic event by the third day. The study results were inconclusive about whether the writing project reduced symptoms of post-traumatic stress since most students reported elevated post-traumatic stress symptoms at the five-month follow-up (Margola et al., 2010).

Not all classmate deaths will be complicated by the level of trauma present in this study, but certainly some will, especially with homicides and accidents that classmates actually witness. Therefore, professionals will want to carefully assess the level of trauma that undergirds childhood and adolescent experiences with loss and ensure appropriate interventions are available. Caregivers must be vigilant to recognize the perceived loss of invincibility and loss of safety that are incumbent with the death of a contemporary in childhood or adolescence.

Pediatric Death in the Professional Community

Death in a young family has a significant impact on those who care for the family, not only in their own social support system but also among professional caregivers. Schoenbine and colleagues (2023) surveyed 337 pediatric oncology professionals from the Children's Oncology Group, a U.S.-based workgroup with more than 10,000 cancer experts in North America, Australia, and New Zealand. They found that most pediatric oncology professionals had attended at least one funeral with slightly more favorable attitudes toward funeral attendance among older professionals. Approximately one in ten respondents disagreed, and approximately half were undecided on the statement, "Funeral attendance respects professional boundaries" (p. 172).

In a qualitative study, researchers asked 23 funeral directors in Northern Ireland about their experiences arranging funerals for families after a parent died from cancer, leaving behind dependent children. Funeral directors reported a heightened level of personal distress since many were parents or grandparents themselves and had difficulty offloading the emotional fallout from working with these families. Funeral directors often reported asking themselves, "What if this happened to my family?" (Hanna et al., 2022, p. 973).

Surveying 210 funeral directors in another part of the world, James et al. (2022) discovered similar emotional difficulties for American professional caregivers. These funeral directors had received little or no professional training for specifically understanding or serving families of pediatric decedents. Nevertheless, respondents felt compelled to remain calm and professional, not permitting their own emotions to cloud their leadership of grieving families. Several interviewees expressed interest in more training from and collaboration with health-care professionals who had pediatric bereavement experience. They also indicated an interest in opportunities to debrief with professionals in the community such as pastors and counselors.

Similarly, in an extensive review of extant literature, Boyle and Bush (2018) found that some pediatric oncology nurses and others who provide care to dying children reported difficulty maintaining professional boundaries with those children's families. Boyle and Bush (2018) reported that changing skill requirements, ineffective coping skills, trouble dealing with challenging family dynamics, and blurred interpersonal boundaries all contributed to the emotional distress experienced by nurses. Blurred professional boundaries were seen to be especially problematic as nurses contacted patients on their days off and engaged in social contact with the patient's family.

Grief after pediatric oncology patient deaths was seen as especially difficult because of the close bond typically forged between professionals, patients, and parents. The death of the child, in turn, caused nurses to wonder if they had done enough, had done the right things at the right times, and had been fully present in the most caring ways (Boyle & Bush, 2018).

Facing the Funeral When a Child Dies

Even though the boy lived for a matter of hours, his life was a treasured gift to his parents, siblings, grandparents, and the wider community of faith and friends where they lived. Because their obstetrician saw structural anomalies in the developing baby at the 15-week sonogram, his parents had spent five months anxiously awaiting his arrival, with a clear understanding that this child's life was precious, that they would care for him deeply for whatever time they had, and that their deep and resonant Catholic faith would see them through the difficulty. However, it was not easy as the infant's dad explained.

In the seventh month of his wife's pregnancy, while he was at a religious retreat and supported by two other fathers who had lost children, the dad reported facing the fury and disappointment of not having been given the child he wanted. In the intervening days, however, he came to realize that the child's life was a gift: "I realized in lamenting what had gone wrong with the pregnancy and what might have been, I was missing the fact that Anthony was alive at that moment" (Gamino, 1999, p. 3). About the interminable waiting, the father wrote, "We did not pray for things to change (e.g., 'a miracle') as did some of our friends. Instead, we prayed for the strength to cope with what was to come" (Gamino, 1999, p. 3).

Anthony lived for only a short time after birth—but long enough to afford time for a baptism—and then peacefully died in the arms of his mom. The ceremonies arranged by this family connected the time-honored rituals of their faith with the needs of their two older children, their extended family, and their network of friends. After spending time with their son in the hospital, in the wee hours of the night, this dad carried his son through the hospital corridors and handed him to the waiting funeral director; it had been imperative for this family that their boy not be taken to the morgue and the hospital staff accommodated the request.

After dressing their son at the funeral home in the burial gown the mom had made while she was pregnant, each immediate family member placed gifts and pictures in the tiny casket, a custom that bereaved families have observed cross-culturally as far back as funerals have been recorded. The siblings, aged eight and four, each placed a favorite toy with their brother, and his dad included a personally written letter of hello and goodbye.

This family had determined in advance that the visitation the night before the funeral mass would be held in their home and people lined up throughout the evening to express their condolences and support. The location seemed only fitting in that every parent expectantly awaits the day they bring their newborn home from the hospital. As the parents drove their son home from the funeral home that afternoon, they followed a route that was anything but a straight line. En route to their home, they made several stops—at the school he would have attended, the parks at which he would have played, the workplaces of his mom and dad, and some of the stores where his family shopped. It was a deliberate procession, but instead of pausing at places that *had been* important to the deceased (as is common in many cultural groups), they stopped at the places that *would have been* important in the child's life and spoke the stories that they longed for their son to hear about the community their family called home.

The traditional Roman Catholic funeral mass the following morning followed a liturgical pattern well known to the family and to many of their friends. The words of the scripture and the strains of the music, along with the cadence of the processional in and out of the church, gave structure to the chaos of this family's grief. "Just as Marla had safely carried Anthony Francis for 38 weeks while he was alive, I now carried him in death," his dad wrote. "I was the only pallbearer he required at the church and at the cemetery" (Gamino, 1999, p. 14).

In what was a horrifying experience at the cemetery to a family already reeling from their loss, the mourners discovered that the grave dug by the workers was too small to accommodate even the tiny casket. As family members were paralyzed in their grief and frozen in their ability to think proactively, a friend from the parish stepped up and used an idle shovel to begin enlarging the small grave so that it was quickly made ready for the burial. Closing the grave was a "community effort," too, with family members and friends joining in the activity of ritual mourning (Gamino, 1999, p. 14). As discussed in Chapter 1, through this simple ritual act, this family and community "walked out what they could not talk out."

Brooten and colleagues (2016) interviewed 63 bereaved parents after their child or infant died in an intensive care unit. They observed that the decision-making process for these parents was stressful and complex as parents worked to integrate culture, beliefs, bereavement experiences, and their financial resources. Some parents expressed regret at not being able to afford to provide an appropriate funeral for their child, and some were particularly glad or sad at the choice they had ultimately made for their child. One parent reported not wanting to see a tiny casket, coupled with concerns about moving from the area and leaving the child's remains behind; another parent expressed deep sadness that financial constraints required cremation rather than transporting the baby to Mexico: "That was what hurt me the most because . . . due to my economic resources he could not be . . . buried. . . . Simply what we did was cremate him" (p. 136).

Creating Ceremonies after Pregnancy Loss

In introducing a grounded theory study of 19 Christian parents following pregnancy loss, Green (2023) observed that even though as many as a quarter of all pregnancies end in loss before birth, there are no culturally prescribed rituals to accompany the experience. For parents of a hoped-for child, the grief is real, the need for social support is intense, and the appreciation is vital of another who understands. Respondents repeatedly voiced that this is a unique grief because of the necessity of facing a loss of one we are "unable to meet" and that communities are generally ill-equipped to offer support—if the community even knows about the loss. Many times, parents and perhaps close family members and friends are the only people aware of the pregnancy and therefore of the loss of that pregnancy (p. 3).

Johnson and Langford (2015) found that clinically significant levels of despair were measurably lower for women who had received a bereavement intervention in the emergency department, when compared to the control group that did not. The intervention included simple activities such as notating the chart so the loss could be acknowledged by health-care team members, referral to a chaplain or connection to the patient's spiritual leader, delivery of a packet of flower seeds for planting at home, and participation in a naming ceremony (p. 495).

Helps and colleagues (2020) reviewed ten reports of patient feedback data related to pregnancy loss and neonatal death from Irish health system–commissioned inquiry reports, concluding, "Bereavement care, as described by families in the ten Irish inquiries was not reliably patient-centred or respectful" (p. 4). Although many parents apparently received no follow-up bereavement care, those who did valued it, at least when the interventions were delivered by staff who were both caring and well trained.

Many pregnancy losses are unexpected with little time to prepare. What seemed to have been a healthy, normal pregnancy suddenly is not, leaving parents reeling from the shock of the unexpected event. As a result, parents cannot be expected to know what they need. Most likely, rituals and ceremonies will need to be executed quickly.

Creating meaningful ceremonies after pregnancy loss is especially challenging because of the potential health complications of the mother who has just delivered a nonviable child, undergone a serious surgical procedure, or who is still in the process of carrying and delivering her deceased child. Moreover, some parents in Green's (2023) study reported their loss was complicated by lack of understanding from health-care professionals and lack of flexibility among the health-care systems caring for them. Although not all parents in the study experienced challenges to their faith, some had significant questions about their beliefs, and their faith communities were sometimes unhelpful.

Naming the baby can be an important part of grief rituals for parents after pregnancy loss in part because such a step helps to make the loss more concrete in a relationship that does not have many living memories attached to it and helps to validate the existence of the baby (Canadian Paediatric Society, 2001; Johnson & Langford, 2015). Parents have often thought of names in advance and can also use the "pet names" they gave to the growing baby; "Little Bump" and "Wee One" are some of the names expectant parents may call their growing baby, even before a gender is known. Even for parents who do not yet know the sex or had not yet decided on the name of their child, some have an intuitive sense about the baby's sex and might decide to choose a birth name based on these or other characteristics. With the help of compassionate caregivers, parents might be interested in having a brief "naming ceremony" with a prayer accompanied by the reading of a favorite text or poem. Lighting a candle as part of this ceremony, with a leader voicing on behalf of those gathered the disappointment from shattered dreams, can be a healing balm to bereaved parents, families, and friends.

In recounting their experiences after the death of an unborn child, some of Green's (2023) respondents expressed they had "mourned until the due date" (p. 58). Some parents found mementos from the hospital—such as memory boxes or baby books—to be helpful, while others created customized reminders. One father enlisted the jeweler who had created their wedding rings to create a ring with an amethyst, the birthstone of the baby's expected birth month. Unfortunately, the stone later fell out of the ring, representing yet another loss.

All of Green's (2023) respondents identified as Christian, and most reported active participation in a faith community at the time of their loss. However, none reported the church offered any kind of formally organized ceremony (although several thought their minister would have cooperated if asked). In the absence of the culturally prescribed rituals that would be expected in the death of an older child, teen, or adult, bereaved parents are left to their own to create a meaningful ceremony. Not all parents would choose a formal ceremony, but in my experience, few are ever given the opportunity to decline.

The Free Methodist Church in Canada (2023) has published useful suggestions for adapting Christian funeral services for miscarriage and stillbirth, suggesting that public prayer can acknowledge the questions facing the family and community, expressing lament and grief while also holding out the hope of faith. Whether in a religiously focused ceremony or not, a naming of the child with perhaps a blessing of the name, lighting of a candle, and presentation of a certificate with the child's name can become an important symbolic reminder of this significant loss (Gamino & Cooney, 2002; Green, 2023).

When my wife and I experienced our first miscarriage a few years before the birth of our first living child, we were at a loss as to what to do. Nowhere in my training had anyone made suggestions about how to memorialize an unborn child after pregnancy loss, and to complicate the matter further, we were traveling at the time of the loss. Fortunately, some friends were close by to provide support. When we returned home, we did the only thing we knew to do instinctively—plant a shrub in this unborn child's memory. Until we moved from that home six years later, the vibrant red flowers of that floribunda "Trumpeter rose" (*rosa trumpeter*) helped us recall the light that expected child had been in our lives. Now three homes later, roses are still an important part of our landscape, and I often wonder whether it is because of the memories attached to that first one. As important as the planting of that rose was, three decades later, we still think periodically about how we would have created additional memorial symbols or events if a caring professional would have guided us. Perhaps colleagues thought, "This is Bill's work; he *knows* what to do," without realizing we can rarely provide such creative care for ourselves.

Community and health-care clergy will often take on leadership roles for families who are thinking about a gathering in memory of their unborn child. Caregivers will want to be ready with suggestions for creating ceremonies or acting out family-only or small-group rituals like the planting of a rosebush or tree. For families without a religious connection, obstetrical practices and hospital emergency departments will want to be ready to assist patients after pregnancy loss with suggestions for resources and links to appropriate websites.

Incorporating Mourning Youth into Memorial Ceremonies

One of the most difficult questions caregivers hear from parents deals with whether and how to include children in funerals. In the years I ran a large family bereavement program in Southern California, I regularly took calls from parents concerned about traumatizing their children if they included them in the funeral. Once I assured them that in nearly every case, it makes sense to include children in the ceremonies, the questions turned to the practical logistics of doing so and how best to involve them in the rituals.

Methven and Warnick (2017) concluded that no child is too young to attend a funeral or memorial if the child has been adequately prepared. Worden (1996) echoed this advice in his report from the Harvard Child Bereavement Study, suggesting that family rituals such as funerals are "important mediators" that affect a child's experience with bereavement. However, for the funeral to have a positive impact, children must be prepared for the experience (p. 21). Furthermore, Worden wrote that when children were not prepared for the funeral experience, they were significantly more likely to be struggling with the experience two years later, including difficulty in discussing the dead parent.

Fristad and colleagues (2001) interviewed 318 young persons (aged 5–17) at 1, 6, 13, and 25 months after the death of a parent. They found that nearly all had attended the parent's visitation, funeral, and burial and that children who did not have those rituals fared less well over time. Attendance at a visitation was associated with better outcomes two years later including lower levels of depression and post-traumatic stress. They found that children derive comfort from familiar items and observances such as the playing of a favorite song.

Similarly, Søfting and colleagues (2016) interviewed 11 children in Norway, finding that the children were grateful to be included in bereavement rituals because it helped them face the reality of the loss and say farewell to the loved one. Being included with the rest of the family, they found, legitimized the children's roles in the family and their experiences with grief.

Worden (1996, pp. 21, 25) noted that 95% of the children in the Boston-area sample attended the funeral but explained that the participation did not lead to later behavioral or emotional problems and that nearly all had positive recollections of the funeral two years after the death.

In a qualitative study of funeral directors from Northern Ireland reflecting on serving families after the deaths of parents, respondents anecdotally reported problems when children were not included in rituals and when parents utilized euphemisms that redefined death (e.g., Mom is a star or an angel). Respondents reported encouraging families to allow children to see their dead parent in the coffin and suggested preparing young children by describing what they would see: the parent would be in a wooden box called a coffin and describing how he or she would be dressed. Respondents described a custom of the casketed body being returned to the family home, which likely makes the involvement of children more central in the ritual of the wake in this cultural practice (Hanna et al., 2022).

Depending on age, young people can be involved in planning family memorial ceremonies including taking part in selecting clothing for the deceased, choosing the casket or urn, designing memorial mementos such as service folders and videos, and offering input on qualities of the deceased to be featured in the eulogy (Hanna et al., 2022; Methven & Warnick, 2017; Worden, 1996).

When young children attend a memorial ceremony, a trusted friend, teacher, or relative outside the immediate family can act as a chaperone for the child. If the service becomes overwhelming, this individual can be responsible for tending to the child so that immediate family can participate in the service with less distraction.

If the casket is open, parents will want to prepare children for that experience and to discuss whether the child wants to view the body; either choice is okay, and children are best served if they are neither forbidden nor forced to see the corpse. Since some children will want to touch the body, it is best for a parent or other caregiver to explain that the hands or face will feel cool to the touch and, assuming the deceased has been embalmed, will likely feel "waxy," a bit like a candle. Describing the experience in as much detail as possible helps bereaved children. Sometimes it is helpful to using sensory language to engage children with the memorial experiences: *smell* the beautiful flowers; *hear* Grandma's favorite hymns/songs being played; *see* Grandpa's favorite necktie that he has on, and so forth.

Many funeral providers have children's rooms set aside equipped with child-sized tables and chairs, art supplies, toys, and videos. Young children will likely find their own comfort objects (such as a beloved teddy bear) to be of help, especially during the period they might be viewing the body of their parent, grandparent, or sibling.

Children often want to place an item such as a letter or piece of artwork in the casket or cremation container. Alternatively, some older children and teens have written poems or letters they read at the memorial ceremony or have someone else read. Children can also be involved in memorial balloon releases at the end of the memorial ceremony or in a different family or small-group ritual. Online retailers offer biodegradable balloons that are preprinted with memorial messages (e.g., "Until we meet again" and "You are not forgotten") as well as balloons that can have personal messages written on them before being released. These memorial ceremonies are especially appropriate for school groups (Palmer, 2021, p. 5).

Clinical Implications

Death and bereavement among children and adolescents is not a topic that is widely discussed in most societies. Caregiving professionals and volunteers have an unusual opportunity to provide education, resources, and support, and the need has never been greater for those interventions than it is today.

Parents and teachers need support, training, and resources when a child in their care is grieving the death of a classmate or sibling. Bereaved parents, grandparents, siblings, and families benefit from a high level of intervention so that they do not think they are walking the bereavement journey alone. This is an especially important opportunity for hospice and hospital professionals, child life specialists, and others who have significant training and experience related to pediatric bereavement.

Most of all, families and communities need help and direction in creating space for children and teens to be involved in funerals for their own parents, siblings, and classmates. Care must be taken to find ways that are age appropriate, but it is imperative that caregivers model healthy grieving practices and discover creative ways to include children in memorial ceremonies.

Reflection and Discussion

- How old were you when you first encountered death personally? Was it the death of a pet, grandparent, parent, sibling, or friend? What do you most recall about the experience and how the adults in your life supported you? How would you change that experience now if you could?
- What are your earliest memories of attending a funeral? Were you included in planning the ceremony, or did you have any part in the service itself? How would you change that?
- What do you see as the greatest challenges in incorporating children in memorial ceremonies? What are your most creative ideas that are not included in this chapter?

References

Boyle, D.A., & Bush, N. J. (2018). Reflections on the emotional hazards of pediatric oncology nursing: Four decades of perspectives and potential. *Journal of Pediatric Nursing*, 40, 63–73. https://doi.org/10.1016/j.pedn.2018.03.007.

Braudt, D.B., Lawrence, E.M., Tilstra, A.M., Rogers, R.G., & Hummer, R.A. (2019). Family socioeconomic status and early life mortality risk in the United States. *Maternal and Child Health Journal*, 23(10), 1382–1391. https://doi.org/10.1007/s10995-019-02799-0.

Brooten, D., Youngblut, J.M., Charles, D., Roche, R., Hidalgo, I., & Malkawi, F. (2016). Death rituals reported by white, Black, and Hispanic parents following the ICU death of an infant or child. *Journal of Pediatric Nursing*, 31(2), 132–140. https://doi.org/10.1016/j.pedn.2015.10.017.

Canadian Paediatric Society. (2001). Guidelines for health care professionals supporting families experiencing a perinatal loss. *Paediatrics & Child Health*, 6 (7), 469–490.

Davies, B. (1988). The family environment in bereaved families and its relationship to surviving sibling behavior. *Children's Health Care*, 17(1), 22–31.

Davies, B. (1999). *Shadows in the sun: Experience of sibling bereavement in childhood*. Brunner/Mazel.

Feigelman, W., Jordan, J.R., & Gorman, B.S. (2011). Parental grief after a child's drug death compared to other death causes: Investigating a greatly neglected bereavement population. *Omega: Journal of Death and Dying*, 63(4), 291–316. https://doi.org/10.2190/OM.63.4.a.

Free Methodist Church in Canada. (2023). Service for miscarriage or stillbirth. https://fmcic.ca/service-for-miscarriage-or-stillbirth/.

Fristad, M.A., Cerel, J., Goldman, M., Weller, E.B., & Weller, R.A. (2001). The role of ritual in children's bereavement. *Omega: Journal of Death and Dying*, 42(4), 321–339. https://doi.org/10.2190/MC87-GQMC-VCDV-UL3U.

Gamino, L.A. (1999). A father's experience of neonatal loss. *The Forum: Association for Death Education and Counseling*, 25(1), 3, 14–15.

Gamino, L.A., & Cooney, A.T. (2002). *When your baby dies through miscarriage or stillbirth*. Augsburg

Gilrane-McGarry, U., & O'Grady, T. (2012). *Forgotten grievers: An exploration of the grief experiences of bereaved grandparents (part 2)*. *International Journal of Palliative Nursing*, 18(4), 179–187. https://doi.org/10.12968/ijpn.2012.18.4.179.

Green, S.F. (2023). *An esoteric grief: A classic grounded theory study on the impact of pregnancy loss* [unpublished bachelor's thesis]. Honors College, Baylor University. https://hdl.handle.net/2104/12208.

Hanna, J.R., McCaughan, E., & Semple, C.J. (2022). Immediate bereavement experiences when a parent of dependent children has died of cancer: Funeral directors' perspectives. *Death Studies*, 46(4), 969–978. https://doi.org/10.1080/07481187.2020.1793433.

Helps, A., O'Donoghue, K., O'Byrne, L., Greene, R., & Leitao, S. (2020). Impact of bereavement care and pregnancy loss services on families: Findings and recommendations from Irish inquiry reports. *Midwifery*, 91, 1–12. https://doi.org/10.1016/j.midw.2020.102841.

Ho, S.-W., & Brotherson, S.E. (2007). Cultural influences on parental bereavement in Chinese families. *Omega: Journal of Death and Dying*, 55(1), 1–25. https://doi.org/10.2190/4293-202L-5475-2161.

Hogan, N.S., & DeSantis, L. (1996). Adolescent sibling bereavement: Toward a new theory. In C.A. Corr & D.E. Balk (Eds.), *Handbook of adolescent death and bereavement* (pp. 173–195). Springer.

James, K., Hawley, B., McCoy, C.R., & Lindley, L.C. (2022). Challenges and opportunities of providing pediatric funeral services: A national survey of funeral professionals. *American Journal of Hospice and Palliative Medicine*, 39(3), 289–294. https://doi.org/10.1177/10499091211019298.

Johnson, O.P., & Langford, R.W. (2015). A randomized trial of a bereavement intervention for pregnancy loss. *Journal of Obstetric, Gynecologic, and Neonatal Nursing*, 44(4), 492–499. https://doi.org/10.1111/1552-6909.12659.

Keesee, N.J., Currier, J.M., & Meymeyer, R.A. (2008). Predictors of grief following the death of one's child: The contribution of finding meaning. *Journal of Clinical Psychology*, 64(10), 1145–1163.

Klass, D., Silverman, P.R., & Nickman, S. (1996). *Continuing bonds: New understandings of grief.* Taylor & Francis.

Margola, D., Facchin, F., Molgora, S., & Revenson, T.A. (2010). Cognitive and emotional processing through writing among adolescents who experienced the death of a classmate. *Psychological Trauma*, 2(3), 250–260. https://doi.org/10.1037/a0019891.

Marshall, B., & Davies, B. (2011). Bereavement in children and adults following the death of a sibling. In R.A. Neimeyer, D.L. Harris, H.R. Winokuer, & G.F. Thornton (Eds.), *Grief and bereavement in contemporary society: Bridging research and practice* (pp. 107–116). Routledge.

McCown, D.E., & Davies, B. (1995). Patterns of grief in young children following the death of a sibling. *Death Studies*, 19(1), 41–53. https://doi.org/10.1080/07481189508252712.

Methven, M., & Warnick, A. (2017). *Preparing children for funerals and memorials.* Canadian Virtual Hospice. https://www.virtualhospice.ca/.

Palmer, J. (2021). *The school bereavement toolkit: A practical guide to supporting children.* Routledge.

Reed, M.L. (1999). *Grandparents cry twice: Help for bereaved grandparents.* Routledge.

Remes, H., Martikainen, P., & Valkonen, T. (2011). The effects of family type on child mortality. *European Journal of Public Health*, 21(6), 688–693. https://doi.org/10.1093/eurpub/ckq159.

Schoenbine, D., Gerhart, J., McLean, K.A., deBettencourt, J., Dadrass, F., Molina, E., Hoerger, M., Alonzi, S., & Kent, P. (2023). Attending patient funerals as a follow-up practice of pediatric oncologists. *Illness, Crisis & Loss*, 31(1), 168–174. https://doi.org/10.1177/10541373211047305.

Søfting, G.H., Dyregrov, A., & Dyregrov, K. (2016). Because I'm also part of the family—Children's participation in rituals after the loss of a parent or sibling: A qualitative study from the children's perspective. *Omega: Journal of Death and Dying*, 73(2), 141–158. https://doi.org/10.1177/0030222815575898.

Song, J., Floyd, F.J., Seltzer, M.M., Greenberg, J.S., & Hong, J. (2010). Long-term effects of child death on parents' health related quality of life: A dyadic analysis. *Family Relations*, 59(3), 269–282. https://doi.org/10.1111/j.1741-3729.2010.00601.x.

Thieleman, K., Cacciatore, J., & Frances, A. (2023). Rates of prolonged grief disorder: Considering relationship to the person who died and cause of death. *Journal of Affective Disorders*, 339, 832–837. https://doi.org/10.1016/j.jad.2023.07.094.

Towers, L. (2022). Knowing what you've got once it's gone: Identifying familial norms and values through the lens of (sibling) bereavement. *Sociology*, 57(5), 1175–1190. https://doi.org/10.1177/00380385221133214.

Udalova, V., Bhatia, V., & Polyakova, M. (2022). Association of family income with morbidity and mortality among US lower-income children and adolescents. *Journal of the American Medical Association*, 328(24), 2422–2430. https://doi.org/10.1001/jama.2022.22778.

United Nations Children's Fund (UNICEF). (2023). *Levels and trends in child mortality.* UNICEF.

Warner, A.B. (1859). Jesus loves me, this I know [hymn lyrics]. https://www.hymnary.com.

Weiss, D.S., & Marmar, C.R. (1997). The Impact of Events Scale–Revised. In J.P. Wilson & T.M. Keane (Eds.), *Assessing psychological trauma and PTSD: A practitioner's handbook* (pp. 399–411). Guilford.

Worden, J.W. (1996). *Children and grief: When a parent dies*. Guilford.

Zunin, L.M., & Zunin, H.S. (1992). *The art of condolence: What to write, what to say, what to do at a time of loss*. HarperCollins.

Chapter 5

Culture, Poverty, and the Cost of Funerals

Throughout history, some individuals have eschewed the pageantry and, likely with it, the cost of funerals. George Washington (1732–1799), the first president of the United States, left strict instructions in his will that "my corpse may be interred in a private manner, without parade or funeral oration" (George Washington & Abraham Lincoln, 2024). Observers have long noted, however, that despite his wishes, the series of events commemorating his death were anything but private and included many parades and orations. Washington's burial at Mount Vernon was attended by his family, household servants, close advisers, and friends, but the nation entered a period of mourning that lasted 69 days from his death on December 14 until his 68th birthday on February 22 (Eliassen, 2023; Reardon, 2023; Tousignant, 2004).

Upon learning of the former president's death, the U.S. Congress meeting in the then-capital city, Philadelphia, immediately adjourned. When the House of Representatives returned the following day, they shrouded the speaker's chair in black, determined that all members would wear black for the remainder of the session, and drafted a funeral plan involving the entire federal government with funeral honors of "solemn and august pageantry" (Eliassen, 2023).

At precisely noon on December 26, the national military funeral procession began at Legislative Hall and continued to German Lutheran Church where a funeral oration was delivered.

> Tolling church bells mingled with the gunfire [of military gun salutes] as musicians performed George Frederick Handel's "Dead March," with the sounds of fifes, muffled drums, and wind instruments (Eliassen, 2023). The interment at Mt. Vernon three days after the president's death had been largely private rather than the grandiose state funeral many heads of state received upon their deaths. However, history demonstrates that common citizens and political leaders alike refused to be denied their opportunities to memorialize the man who was already being referred to widely as the nation's "father."
>
> (Lim, 2023)

DOI: 10.4324/9781003353010-6

In part inspired by Washington's funeral, the U.S. Army has developed a 138-page plan for state funerals which is customized by each president shortly after election (Hoy, 2013; Tousignant, 2004).

Funerals for political leaders and entertainment celebrities are typically grandiose affairs costing thousands if not millions of dollars. Funerals for celebrities such as recording artist Whitney Houston, described in Chapter 8, can boast thousands of people in attendance. The funeral for "King of Pop" Michael Jackson had more than 17,000 in attendance in addition to uncountable thousands on the Los Angeles streets surrounding Staples Center. What shocked many around the world, however, was the cost for the 2009 funeral—more than US$2.3 million including $35,000 for burial garments, $21,455 for the funeral "repast" (meal) after the service, and $16,000 for flowers. These costs were paid by Jackson's estate and the Jackson family, but the city of Los Angeles also incurred costs exceeding $1 million for police and crowd control (Michaels, 2009).

Although the average person's funeral lacks the complexity and the cost of these celebrity ceremonies, questions remain about equitable costs for rituals. Are those costs evidence of a greedy funeral profession that preys on the emotions of vulnerable and distraught families who are grieving the death of a loved person? Are the solutions that have been frequently touted as "simple" really simple, or have many families and communities simply jettisoned one kind of ceremony and replaced it with something even more extravagant? How do those expenditures fit into a needy world, especially when, at least at first blush, it appears those with the fewest resources arrange the most traditional, and theoretically most costly, ceremonies? What are caregiving professionals and interested others to do to protect the most vulnerable among them in the face of the so-called high cost of dying? These and many questions like them are the subject of this chapter.

From Funeral Criticism to Government Regulation

Formal criticism of funeral directors and funeral customs has been ongoing for at least a century with calls for reform of the American funeral industry dating to the 1920s (Laderman, 2005). The University of Chicago Press published Quincy Dowd's (1921) study of burial customs and prices in many of the world's largest nations, concluding that the poor were often disadvantaged by the predatory pricing of funerals. The overarching conclusion of Dowd, seconded by Mark's (1923) review in the *American Journal of Sociology*, was that the poor of the United States were more subject to exploitation because of lax state regulation and that "the simple and inexpensive disposal of the dead is in harmony with social welfare, and that all classes of society in America need to be educated to this point of view" (Mark, 1923, p. 505).

In his survey of American funeral history in the 20th century, Laderman (2005) noted that there were many groups of ministers in the 1930s and beyond who led the criticism of death practices as they were observed in the early decades of the 20th century. In one example, Laderman noted an article by Tigner (1937), which outlined the conclusions drawn by a group of New York ministers about the increasingly large role funeral directors were playing in funeral rituals (while clergy seemed of secondary importance), as well as their criticism that the worship of the body was a pagan practice rather than one borne of historic Christian values and theology. The ministers' eight-point recommendation report, published in the *Christian Century*, called for simplicity including such instructions as disposing of the body quickly, keeping the casket closed to avoid worship of the body, and avoiding music and singing because of its tendency to be inconsistent with the need for quietness a funeral demands (Tigner, 1937, p. 1264, as cited in Laderman, 2005, p. 63). Laderman went on to suggest that this criticism was far from isolated, citing examples from the Federal Council of Churches in the 1940s and Roman Catholics in the early 1960s.

By the early 1960s, criticism of funerals had reached a fever pitch. British author Evelyn Waugh (1948) had published a satirical novel about a fictional funeral home and cemetery called Whispering Glades that bore striking resemblance to California's Forest Lawn, which Waugh had visited. The satire of Waugh, however, proved to be light compared to the satirical exposé produced by another British-born journalist, Jessica Mitford (1963). Unlike Waugh's depiction that seemed to exaggerate the mundane elements of funeral service, *The American Way of Death* purported to represent the experiences of thousands of unaware consumers who had been duped by the American funeral industry. The criticisms included the selling of expensive caskets, burial vaults, and limousines when a simple cremation would suffice.

Mitford's book was an instant bestseller and would likely have been more effective if not for an accident of timing. A few months after *The American Way of Death* was published, President John F. Kennedy was assassinated. People in the United States and around the world were riveted to their televisions to view a state funeral in all its dignity, honor, and pageantry (Laderman, 2005). An attempt to help assuage a nation in grief, Kennedy's funeral displayed all of the grandeur that had caused George Washington to wince nearly two centuries earlier.

The rising tide of criticism, however, did eventually lead the U.S. Federal Trade Commission in the mid-1970s to conduct investigations and open hearings to study the reports of misdeeds and price gouging in the funeral industry. In the commission's staff report and recommendations, staff was highly critical of American funeral trade practices, finding that consumers had been required to pay for items of services they did not choose or use, such as embalming, viewing, and family limousines. The staff report criticized the funeral industry:

> This high level of consumer ignorance is due in part to the continued efforts of the funeral industry to minimize the ability of consumers to obtain meaningful itemized price information in advance or at the time funeral arrangements are being made.
>
> (U.S. Federal Trade Commission, 1978, p. 381)

After adoption of the Funeral Rule in 1984, the Federal Trade Commission revisited the rule with hearings in 1994 and 2004, providing some clarifications but reaffirming the original trade rule. Later, the U.S. Federal Trade Commission (2007) published a list of "core rights" to which every funeral consumer could expect to be entitled. These rights included such items as buying only the items desired, obtaining pricing information over the phone, getting a written statement of decisions made before payment is rendered, and the ability to use a casket or urn purchased somewhere other than the funeral home (p. 2).

Interestingly, the commission's staff report from 1978 quoted several business and economics professors who surmised that the recommended rule would allow consumers to choose more freely because providing price information would cause funeral homes to compete on price. "With the advent of price-oriented behavior and a concomitant rise in the level of competition," staff wrote, "consumers will be able to avoid unnecessary funeral expenses" (U.S. Federal Trade Commission, 1978, p. 508).

Despite frequent media reports comparing funeral costs, investigative stories on the unfair and unethical practices, and the ongoing efforts of funeral critics who decry the high cost of death and consistently suggest that the poor are most vulnerable to the funeral industry's predatory practices (Slocum & Carlson, 2011), the highest priced funeral providers in virtually every community continue to thrive with seemingly little progress made by low-cost operators (Hoy, 2013, 2022). The role of culture and tradition, especially among some of the low-resource communities that critics promise to "protect," has proven refractory to reform. Apparently, significant numbers of people living in poverty in the United States prefer elaborate funerals rather than the simplified versions researchers and critics seem to believe should be normative for everyone.

The United Kingdom, through its Competition and Markets Authority (CMA), enacted rules in 2021 that are similar in scope to those in the United States. From 2019 through 2021, the CMA conducted an investigation and sought comments related to funeral practices in the United Kingdom, issuing its final Funerals Market Investigation Order 2021 on April 15, 2021. The order required funeral directors and crematorium operators to provide price information to consumers and competitors through a Standardised Price List that would allow price comparison between providers and to disclose business relationships (such as corporate ownership). Like the General Price List in the United States, the United Kingdom's Standardised Price List must include itemized prices for items such as an attended funeral (funeral director and mourners present), an unattended funeral (called a "direct burial" in the United States), embalming, and vehicles (United Kingdom Consumer Protection, 2021)

The Australian Competition and Consumer Commission (2023) has taken a less centralized approach to funeral regulation than in the United States or United Kingdom, declaring that business practices must be fair and that consumers must not be misled but largely leaving pricing regulation to states and territories. The Australian Competition and Consumer Commission's (2021) report on funeral competition considered the results of 572 respondents (72% who had recently arranged a funeral) and found that pricing disclosure was not always clear, with 13% of consumers reporting they did not get pricing information in their first meeting with the funeral director and 44% reporting they had to ask for pricing disclosure (pp. 7–8).

The survey also found evidence that some funeral service contracts included unfair terms such as punitive interest rates and late fees. Moreover, the commission found that customers were sometimes misled by false claims of local ownership by corporate operators, a significant finding in that one-third of all funeral providers in Australia are owned by two corporate organizations (pp. 4, 11–12). The commission also found some evidence that prearrangement contracts were not always fulfilled as promised and that some funeral providers "bundled" services and products, and alleged these practices reduce price transparency and competition (p. 14).

The Australian states of New South Wales, Victoria, and most recently, Queensland have enacted state-level laws to protect funeral consumers. These laws require various levels of price disclosure and licensure or registration by funeral directors. Pricing regulation in New South Wales is of importance since more than one-third of Australians live within the state and it ranks as the fastest growing Australian state (New South Wales Government, 2023). New South Wales's funeral price disclosure laws enacted in 2019 requires funeral providers to disclose specific items on a price list, to make those prices available to consumers in advance, and to disclose relationships with other entities such as corporate holding companies (New South Wales Government, 2019).

Despite growing government regulation of funeral providers, funeral consumer groups around the world insist that price regulation does not go far enough in protecting consumers. Advocates for funeral reform have repeatedly suggested that lax enforcement by regulators and low financial penalties provide little incentive for providers to comply with the law (Slocum & Carlson, 2011).

Funeral Poverty and a Kenyan Solution

As a term that emerged in the early 21st century, "funeral poverty" is broadly defined to include an inability to pay for funeral costs to create the ceremonies desired and the economic impact that creates (such as indebtedness). These elements are coupled with the negative emotional impact these phenomena have on the individual's experience of bereavement. Across the social and behavioral sciences globally, increasing attention and research in recent years have focused on funeral poverty (Corden & Hirst, 2015; Valentine & Woodthorpe, 2014).

The Luo of rural western Kenya provide an illustrative example of how funerals and poverty often intersect. A few years after Straw to Bread, a U.S.-based development organization, began working with Bethlehem Home (its counterpart in Sigoti, Kenya), a team of professors and students from Baylor University visited the project in May 2012 to spend three weeks working together. Upon arrival, the leader of the local community, Habil Ogola, explained to Dr. Lisa Baker, the pediatrician-director of Straw to Bread, that his community was facing a significant conundrum. The AIDS epidemic had decimated the community, as it had many sub-Saharan African communities, leaving a largely absent middle generation.

Like in previous years, the death rate was high, and funerals were culturally vital to Ogola's people. When a member of the Luo tribe dies, custom dictates that the funeral involves a Friday afternoon to Saturday noon funeral observance, often attended by 200 or 300 family members, relatives, and friends. The "traditions of the elders" called for the body to be brought back to the family homestead; therefore, in addition to the hospital mortuary fee for embalming, there was almost always a fee for transportation from the not-so-close hospital where the body would have been taken, even if the death occurred at home.

At the hour for Friday afternoon tea, family and friends began to gather for the beginning of the funeral ceremony. Specialized catering equipment like canopies, tables, chairs, cooking vessels, and serving utensils were all needed in addition to a large quantity of meat, vegetables, and ugali, the maize-based doughy cake that is a staple of the Luo diet. With so many people to feed and so many details to arrange, the common option for families was to hire a caterer. Along with transportation and the traditional undertaking costs at the hospital, the cost was high for a culturally appropriate funeral meal, often causing families to sell off a portion of their cropland to pay the bill. That decision, in turn, caused even more hardship on the farming families who were often at the edge of starvation in their subsistence economy.

Nevertheless, even facing abject poverty, most refused to forgo their generations-old cultural practices to choose less costly options regardless of how many global economists had advised them to do so. Although there had been many efforts during the height of the global AIDS crisis to simplify funerals, Case and colleagues (2013) noted that in South Africa, as was the case with many of its sub-Saharan African neighbors, efforts had failed. As had been observed among the Luo on the Kenyan Nyakach Plateau, the researchers found that funerals in South Africa were elaborate and expensive with a family shouldering the costs for a coffin, funeral tents, and entertainment expenses.

As the Luo of the Kenyan Nyakach expressed their concerns to their American visitors who listened to their priorities, the Kenyans suggested a possible solution. Their question was simple. Would it be feasible for the American group to provide seed money to help them begin their own funeral catering business? With some collaborative research conducted while the team was in the community those weeks, it was found that an investment of US$1,200 would provide equipment as well as training for a dozen individuals from the community who would become catering professionals. Each of the women chosen represented one of the existing business groups, which effectively spread the potential profits among all segments of the community.

Within a few months, the business was running, paying the workers who delivered and set up the equipment and the caterers who cooked and served the meals, while retaining enough earnings to expand and replace equipment as needed. What was unique about the funeral business was its gift each month to the community's school for orphans and a food and agriculture program for needy elders—a gift made not from the leftovers of profits but from the top of revenues. The organization's commitment to community was selfless even from its outset.

The model seemed simple enough. When a family in the community had little or no ability to pay, the community's catering business would step in and provide the services at little or no cost. When bereaved individuals and families had the ability to pay, they would pay an amount that was probably still well below market rates but would help the funeral catering business to make a modest profit on its work after paying workers employed from the community. When individuals from outside the Bethlehem Home community (neighboring towns) requested the services of the funeral catering business, they would pay an amount competitively priced with similar services in those communities. The people overseeing the development of the funeral catering business would not try to undercut their competitors, but they would seek to provide a comparable or superior service at a fair price, always bathed with their own Christian compassion (Hoy, 2013).

Within a few years, the U.S.-based nonprofit had helped the Bethlehem Home community build, equip, and staff a small hospital and members of the Straw to Bread team continued to work in the community every year. Then, government inspectors noted that the hospital must provide its own mortuary, and the idea was born to build a free-standing funeral home that would meet government requirements and likely become an option for families on the highly traveled highway a few kilometers from the hospital. Community members would be recruited to complete the government-required training program for morticians and to work as attendants and hosts. Like with the catering business begun a few years earlier, the funeral home would offer its services at a competitive price, but if a family with a known financial need was being served, a sliding scale, much like that used by many clinical readers of this volume, would make sure every family could be served at a price they could afford.

The COVID-19 pandemic delayed the opening and full operation of the funeral home, but within two years of beginning service to the community, the business was successful in the same way as its funeral catering business had been, employing people in the community in serving their neighbors and families from nearby towns while making a reasonable profit. Unlike the other hospital mortuaries where families are expected to pay fees before discussing arrangements, the Bethlehem Home funeral organization offers Christian hospitality, inviting newly bereaved families to first sit down with a cup of tea and a funeral home employee to share stories. A small open-air chapel in the funeral home courtyard provides a shaded location for families to gather with their loved ones and say goodbye, a feature other hospital mortuaries in the area do not offer to families.

The funeral home was built on a busy highway between two larger towns but is located on lands that border two feuding tribes who have historically fought over possession of the land. The leaders of the Bethlehem Home made the unprecedented move to hire not only employees from their own community but also from the community some would consider their "enemy." The result has been that the funeral home, in addition to becoming a haven where the dead are cared for and where grieving families find comfort, has transformed into a center for community reconciliation, healing, and forgiveness.

The funeral home has its own water source. Upon realizing that members of the community were dying from lack of water, Bethlehem Home's leaders decided to make their water freely available to the community. Although government regulations require a locked security wall around the funeral home property, leaders installed a water tap near the road outside the walls and have invited community members to take what they need for their own families.

Poverty and Funerals among African Americans

Many bereavement professionals, funeral directors, and clergy in my research have anecdotally observed that families who often are most at risk because of poverty are the very families who frequently arrange elaborate ceremonies. Acknowledging that one in five African American families lives below the poverty line, the grounded theory study conducted in 2019–2022 sought to understand from bereaved families, clergy, funeral directors, and health-care professionals what families might most value as they make funeral choices. Guiding the study was a desire to understand how low-resource families fund the choices made to honor their loved one's lives in culturally meaningful ways despite the significant financial constraints they face. Several key themes emerged in the interviews with this wide diversity of bereaved individuals and the professionals who care for them (Hoy, 2022).

Results in this study of the interplay between funeral choice, cultural customs, and economic means found that bereaved families place a high value on spiritual truth, meaningful music integrated into the ceremony, an emphasis on declared scripture, and preaching in the context of the entire gathered (spiritual) community. These services are most frequently led by a member of the clergy, and most often, it is a pastor well known to the deceased or to at least the family. The common use of the term "homegoing" to describe these services is an example of the spiritual focus of these ceremonies, a finding that echoes the research of Na and Hoy (2015). The unique aspects of African American homegoing ceremonies are explored more fully in Chapter 8 of this volume.

Also echoing the earlier research of Na and Hoy (2015) is the finding that gathering of family and friends in the presence of the corpse is vital. Clearly, embalming of the body, additional preparation of the deceased for presentation to the public, and the purchase of a casket add significant costs to the funeral invoice. Without question, a direct cremation—as recommended by many ministers outside of African American communities in the first half of the 20th century—would be a far less expensive way to dispose of the corpse. However, even for African American families who struggle with economic security, the direct cremation is rarely chosen. In every city where I interviewed African American funeral directors and funeral home owners, there was a plethora of lower cost providers available to families, yet it seems African American families rarely chose to utilize their services (Hoy, 2022). Buchanan and Gabriel (2015) found a similar reticence to embrace cremation, especially among older religious African Americans, though younger people seem to be more accepting. In my research, I have consistently found, however, that even when African American families choose cremation as the mode of final disposition, that arrangement is frequently preceded by a visitation with the casketed, embalmed body and frequently, a church funeral. Sometimes a ceremonial (rental) casket is available, but I have found rarely do African American families choose to utilize such an option.

In some cases, clergy interviewed felt there was a strong preference for African American families to choose a funeral home that is owned by and specifically caters to other African Americans. One clergyman explained, "I know the Black firms in town are not cheap. But my people are going to use a Black-owned business whenever they can. And besides that, African American funeral directors just make the body look better than White funeral homes do."

Several respondents of the African American funeral choice study explained the meanings behind their choices when they had recently arranged a funeral service for a loved one. There was significant concern that the body be treated with dignity in death, even if the person's life had been subject to significant racism and the indignities of the health-care system. Respondents also frequently mentioned the desire to pay tribute to the deceased. As one bereaved mother described her family's decisions, "We wanted to give him a final gift even if we had to pay for it later."

African American clergy pointed to the desire of many families to choose a funeral home with a contemporary, matching, professional automotive fleet because it offers a point of pride to the family at the funeral service. Making sure that all family members ride in a limousine requires funeral directors to operate several cars for that purpose. One funeral home owner said three or four family limousines on a single service is not uncommon in her community even though families pay an additional fee for each of these cars. One clergyperson suggested that some people in his church "want to look rich at the funeral even if they don't have the money to pay the rent."

One mother whose divorced adult daughter died from COVID-19 in the midst of the pandemic expressed significant regret at having been financially unable to do everything she wanted to do for the service. She arranged a brief visitation using a simple casket at the African American–owned funeral home in her community, followed by cremation. Ironically, the Statement of Goods and Services she produced as evidence of the amount she paid represented an amount almost double what the cost would have been at a competing funeral home a few blocks away but that was not owned by an African American businessman. The bereaved mother reported choosing the funeral home she did without comparison shopping and falsely assuming that the White-owned business would have cost even more.

Bereaved family members and caregiving professionals indicated a diversity of sources for paying funeral costs, though all of the African American funeral homes surveyed require costs to be paid in full before the services are held. Funeral homes offer "donation pages" wherein community members can make contributions to the funeral account of a bereaved family, and a number of families and professionals pointed to crowdsourcing websites where funds have been raised. There are some government assistance programs for indigent funeral care, though these seem to be limited in the United States. More frequently, there are funds available to pay portions of funeral expenses through the Federal Emergency Management Administration (FEMA) for deaths related to COVID-19 and for various victims of violent crimes funds. Sometimes community members simply get together and hold a car wash or a bake sale to help out a friend in need.

Proposed Alternatives to the High Cost of Funerals

Members of some associations of funeral directors pledge themselves to take care of the poor within their means. The international voluntary association Selected Independent Funeral Homes (2012) requires its members to subscribe to its Code of Good Practice, which states in its second provision, "To make services available in as wide a range of price categories as necessary to meet the needs of all segments of our community, and to affirmatively extend to everyone the right to inspect and freely consider them all" (n.p.). Similarly, the International Order of the Golden Rule (2020), another voluntary association of independently owned funeral homes, requires its members to abide by the second standard in its code of ethics: "We pledge ourselves to serve any deserving family in time of need, regardless of monetary consideration" (n.p.).

The pledges of the independent funeral home associations are significant in that Slocum (2017) found that independent funeral home prices were significantly lower than those at funeral homes owned by New York Stock Exchange–traded Service Corporation International (SCI) in the ten U.S. metropolitan areas Slocum surveyed. Comparing the median prices on the General Price List for three typical service types, the study found that SCI-owned funeral firms charged 72% more for simple (direct) cremation, 50% more for direct burial, and 47% more for full-service funerals. The study compared prices among 103 independently owned funeral firms and compared them to 35 competing SCI-owned firms in Georgia, Arizona, California, Colorado, Indiana, Minnesota, Pennsylvania, New Jersey, Washington, and the District of Columbia.

Although these data are compelling on their face, caution is advised in interpreting them because the General Price Lists for SCI firms were collected in 2017 while the price lists for independent firms were collected in 2015 and then adjusted by the rate of inflation in effect during those years. These adjustments appear to be generous since the National Funeral Directors Association (2021) recent price survey demonstrated that during 2016–2021, American funeral prices rose at a rate below the rate of inflation. In the study period, the median cost of adult funerals increased 6.6% and the median cost of funerals with cremation increased 11.3%, while the overall rate of inflation was 13.98% for the same period.

Many funeral homes provide free or deeply reduced cost packages in the cases of deaths of children and adolescents. Health-care social workers and chaplains typically know which local funeral providers are willing to work with families within their ability to pay, and nearly every clergyperson interviewed in my research tells of a time a local funeral director provided complete services at little or no cost to a needy family. Most caregiving professionals interviewed indicated that it would be an independent, usually family-owned funeral firm in the community who could best be relied on to care for an indigent family. One such firm's owner reported that the funeral home's accounting audit discovered that the dollar value of discounted or complimentary funerals that year (2019) had exceeded the combined annual salary and benefits of the two co-owners.

Many American and Canadian funeral and cremation providers require full payment or guaranteed life insurance assignment before services are completed; a few firms will reschedule services that are not yet paid for. Other funeral homes provide a limited amount of time for families to pay expenses and, as a result, see their accounts receivables balloon with uncollected invoices that far exceed the time given to families to pay. Many of these firms also have funding partners that allow families to arrange credit to make payments for the funeral they arrange, perhaps over 24–48 months, and these firms also accept credit cards as payment. But as one funeral home owner described the dilemma, "Once the funeral is over, our only recourse against a family who does not pay is to sue them. I'm not like a bank that can just repossess a car."

What is unknown is the amount of unsecured debt families are incurring to purchase the options they choose. These choices are not unlike other large consumer purchases such as automobiles, furniture, and major appliances where individuals incur thousands of dollars in debt as they pay for these items over time, an option that often results in the purchase of luxury items that a financially savvy observer might consider economically unwise.

Nevertheless, debt on these big-ticket items like cars, furniture, and funerals can carry high interest rates and stiff late-payment penalties. Social economists have long noted that the cultural customs of individuals with inability to pay, paired with an inability to take advantage of early-payment discounts, have led to a continuing gap between rich and poor when it comes to funeral expenditures. Growing levels of funeral poverty have caused some to call for increased social benefit programs similar to nationalized health coverage and even state-run funeral service organizations (Drakeford, 1998; Fan & Zick, 2004; Fletcher & McGowan, 2021; Valentine & Woodthorpe, 2014).

In a provocative pilot study, Valentine and Woodthorpe (2014) examined the funeral social welfare policies in 12 nations, 4 each from 3 typologies: liberal regimes, corporatist regimes, and social democratic regimes. Denmark, the Netherlands, Norway, and Sweden, characterized in the study authors' research as "social democratic regimes," were found to provide significant funeral benefits for most or all residents of the state, funded generally by universal taxes. Some of these benefits were in the form of universal grants, while others utilized some type of means-testing formula to calculate how much state support was needed to supplement the deceased's assets. In all four countries, state funds were available for those who were in need of additional support (p. 527).

Several social economy scholars and researchers have noted what Kearl (1989) summarized: "The tendency of lower-class families to provide their members in death the dignity . . . that they did not receive in life has contributed to the growth of a multibillion-dollar industry" (p. 283).

Funerals in the Nonprofit Sector

Charities and organizations to which the deceased (or family) belong have sometimes been a source for funeral funding. Labor unions, clubs, and faith communities occasionally provide funds to bereaved families on a means-tested basis or simply as a benefit of membership in the organization. One California funeral director reported that the large Cambodian population in his community funded funerals through a "fellowship fund" by paying the cost of a chapel funeral service and cremation in a cherry or maple casket for every dues-paying member of the community association.

Religious organizations have often operated nonprofit hospitals and cemeteries, but only in recent years have religious groups attempted to operate funeral homes, businesses that have historically been for-profit organizations. Across the United States during the middle of the 20th century, memorial associations arose to address what their advocates regularly called the high costs of dying. Slocum and Carlson (2011, p. 23) called for a growth in consumer-friendly nonprofit memorial associations and low-cost nonprofit funeral homes even though they suggested some state laws would prohibit such an approach.

One nonprofit funeral home in the northeastern United States operates with the encouragement and support of a large religious community. Like other nonprofit entities, it is required to report its revenues, expenses, net income (or loss), and assets to the U.S. Internal Revenue Service (IRS). A survey of this organization's IRS form 990 from 2016 through 2021 revealed that in its most recent year, its total revenues were approximately US$3.5 million, though operating expenses exceeded revenues by about a quarter-million dollars. Expenses recorded on the 2021 Form 990 indicated that the organization paid its executive officers and key employees similarly to owners of independent funeral homes in the region. The organization spent approximately 44% of expenses on salaries, payroll taxes, and employee benefits, 12% on automobile expense, 10% on occupancy and office/technology expense, and slightly more than 10% on advertising and promotion. The organization also paid nearly 5% of total expenses for external management and accounting services.

Across six years surveyed, the organization lost a cumulative US $350,000, an amount that had to be supplemented by fundraising activities and cash already on hand. The six-year loss would have exceeded $600,000 if not for a substantial positive earnings year in 2020, the year in which the COVID-19 pandemic began. As a nonprofit entity, the organization is not responsible for federal or state income taxes and has the opportunity to make direct appeals to the community for support to subsidize its services. This organization also received substantial gifts and grants to make its initial capital investment for property, facilities, and equipment. If not for those tax-deductible gifts when the organization began, it would show a much broader financial loss including the mortgage principal and interest payments it did not have to pay because of the initial fundraising appeal.

The funeral business is a high-cost business with substantial required outlays to provide the staff, facilities, and equipment to be available to bereaved families around the clock, but it has not proven to be a highly profitable business. A decade ago, many other industries including hospices, dental offices, educational service businesses, and accounting firms were demonstratively at least as profitable or more profitable than funeral service businesses (Hoy, 2013, pp. 142–145). Current analyses indicate those facts remain unchanged, and interviews with funeral directors and association representatives point to a shrinking of profit margins over recent years rather than an expansion of them.

Moreover, the assumption that nonprofit organization and low-cost services go together is not borne out by the data. One memorial association in the northwestern region of the United States regularly conducts price surveys. Since the association both contracts with local providers and owns its own nonprofit funeral home, it seemed important to compare General Price Lists between several of the for-profit competitors and the nonprofit. Because the Federal Trade Commission mandates the language of the General Price List, the comparison of prices is easy and straightforward.

Although many consumer advocates would assume the nonprofit association-owned funeral home's prices would be significantly lower priced than its rivals, exactly the opposite is what was found to be true. Prices for direct cremation ranged from less than US$600 to over $4,000. Thirteen providers, most of which were for-profit firms, quoted prices lower than the nonprofit. Four funeral homes, including one other nonprofit, offered a complete traditional burial service at a lower price than the nonprofit memorial association's firm. One for-profit entity in the community disclosed lower prices on nearly every item the Federal Trade Commission mandates on the price list, and the nonprofit firm's price was more than double on at least two of those items.

Funeral poverty remains a thorny issue for individuals, families, communities, governments, and society at large. The emotion of early bereavement, especially when the death was unexpected or traumatic, paired with cultural expectations surrounding funerals in the lowest-resource communities, will continue to challenge efforts to make substantial progress on reform. Conversations within families and community groups about what is appropriate along with efforts to increase access to advance planning programs are important. Likewise, consumers educating themselves in advance, thinking through options, shopping carefully for providers in advance, and considering ways to lower costs are important tactics (Potts, 2021).

Clinical Implications

Clinicians in end-of-life settings such as hospices, skilled nursing facilities, and hospital critical care units will want to know what options are available in the community, always keeping in mind that what caregiving professional thinks is a "smart, inexpensive choice" might not fulfill a bereaved family's cultural expectations. Patience and dialogue are essential as is knowing what options, resources, and benefit programs are available in the community.

In any setting, clinicians and other caregivers must be alert to funeral poverty that might be the result of decisions related to "keeping up appearances" and "saving face" in extended family and community. At the same time, caregiving professionals must remain alert that some individuals see consumer debt as a reasonable concession to having the things in life that might not be available for cash. Funerals are not the only large purchases for which families incur debt, and caregivers need to remain alert to the balance between cultural choices and economic resources.

Moreover, caregivers will want to always be ready to advocate for those they serve who struggle in low-resource settings and want to choose affordable ceremonies that help them start the meaning-creation process without the extravagance that a cultural custom might suggest is needed. When bereaved individuals and families make decisions not in concert with community expectations, these individuals will likely require extra support in the bereavement process.

Reflection and Discussion

- What do you think about cultural customs that potentially create poverty? How do you think your opinion is based on your own set of values that might actually demonstrate your own inability to be culturally attuned?

- Should governments include funeral benefits as a "safety net" program that helps defray the cost of a funeral? If so, how much should the government contribute? If you disagree with government intervention, what is the source of your opposition?
- Have you talked with your family about your funeral plans including a discussion of what each person wants and why they find that meaningful? Based on your cultural and family customs and your research in your community, how much do you think is a reasonable amount to spend?

References

Australian Competition and Consumer Commission. (2021). Funeral services sector report: Competition and consumer issues. https://www.accc.gov.au/.

Australian Competition and Consumer Commission. (2023). Funeral services. https://www.accc.gov.au/.

Buchanan, T., & Gabriel, P. (2015). Race differences in acceptance of cremation: Religion, Durkheim, and death in the African American community. *Social Compass*, 62(1), 22–42. https://doi.org/10.1177/0037768614560949.

Case, A., Garrib, A., Menendez, A., & Olgiati, A. (2013). Paying the piper: The high cost of funerals in South Africa. *Economic Development and Cultural Change*, 62(1), 1–20. https://doi.org/10.1086/671712.

Corden, A., & Hirst, M. (2015). The meaning of funeral poverty: An exploratory study. (Working Paper WP 2668). Social Policy Research Unit, University of York. https://www.mariecurie.org.uk/globalassets/media/documents/policy/policy-publications/march-2016/meaning-of-funeral-poverty-exploratory-study.pdf.

Dowd, Q.L. (1921). *Funeral management and costs*. University of Chicago Press.

Drakeford, M. (1998). Last rights? Funerals, poverty and social exclusion. *Journal of Social Policy*, 27(4), 507–524. https://doi.org/10.1017/S0047279498005376.

Eliassen, M. (2023). Mourning George Washington. Digital Encyclopedia, George Washington Presidential Library at Mount Vernon. https://www.mountvernon.org/library/.

Fan, J.X., & Zick, C.D. (2004). The economic burden of health care, funeral, and burial expenditures at the end of life. *Journal of Consumer Affairs*, 38(1), 35–55. https://doi.org/10.1111/j.1745-6606.2004.tb00464.x.

Fletcher, S., & McGowan, W. (2021). The state of the UK funeral industry. *Critical Social Policy*, 41(2), 249–269. https://doi.org/10.1177/0261018320932279.

George Washington and Abraham Lincoln. (2024). [Digital file.] Online Collection, University of Michigan Library. https://clements.umich.edu/exhibit/death-in-early-america/washington-lincoln/.

Haneman, V.J. (2021). Funeral poverty. *University of Richmond Law Review*, 55(2), 387–445.

Hoy, W.G. (2013). *Do funerals matter? The purposes and practices of death rituals in global perspective*. Routledge.

Hoy, W.G. (2022, April 22). *African American funeral choice: The role of cultural customs and economic means*. Paper presented at the Association for Death Education and Counseling, St. Louis, MO.
International Order of the Golden Rule. (2020). Standards of ethical conduct. https://www.ogr.org/ethical-standards-ogr.
Kearl, M.C. (1989). *Endings: A sociology of death and dying*. Oxford University Press.
Laderman, G. (2005). *Rest in peace: A cultural history of death and the funeral home in twentieth-century America*. Oxford University Press.
Lim, R. (2023). Father of his country. Digital Encyclopedia, George Washington Presidential Library at Mount Vernon. https://www.mountvernon.org/library/.
Mark, M.L. (1923). Review of *Funeral management and costs* by Quincy L. Dowd. *American Journal of Sociology*, 28(4), 504–505. https://doi.org/10.1086/213525.
Michaels, S. (2009, November 12). Michael Jackson's funeral cost $1m. *The Guardian*. https://www.theguardian.com.
Mitford, J. (1963). *The American way of death*. Simon & Schuster.
Na, Y., & Hoy, W.G. (2015, April 22). *Examining video to clarify African American funeral experiences*. Paper presented at the Association for Death Education and Counseling, San Antonio, TX.
National Funeral Directors Association. (2021, November 4). 2021 NFDA General Price List study shows funeral costs not rising as fast as rate of inflation. https://www.nfda.org/news/.
New South Wales Government. (2019, September 3). New regulation gives funeral pricing transparency for bereaved consumers. https://www.nsw.gov.au/news/.
New South Wales Government. (2023). Key facts about NSW. https://www.nsw.gov.au/.
Potts, L. (2021, December 1). Eight tips for funeral planning: How to make smart decisions and arrangements. American Association for Retired Persons. https://www.aarp.org.
Reardon, J.M. (2023). Who is the funeral really for? *American Funeral Director*, 146(6), 40–42.
Selected Independent Funeral Homes. (2012). Our code of good practice. https://www.selectedfuneralhomes.org/Consumers.
Slocum, J. (2017). Death with dignity? A report on SCI/Dignity Memorial high prices and refusal to disclose those prices. Consumer Federation of America. https://consumerfed.org/funerals/.
Slocum, J., & Carlson, L. (2011). *Final rights: Reclaiming the American way of death*. Upper Access Books.
Tigner, H.S. (1937). A foray into funeral customs. *Christian Century*, 54(41), 1263–1265.
Tousignant, M. (2004, June 10). Two hundred years of presidential funerals. *Washington Post*. https://www.washingtonpost.com/archive/.
United Kingdom Consumer Protection. (2021). Funerals market investigation order 2021. https://www.gov.uk/business/consumer-protection.
U.S. Federal Trade Commission. (1978). *Funeral industry practices: Final staff report to the Federal Trade Commission and proposed trade regulation rule (16 CFR Part 453)*. U.S. Government Printing Office.

U.S. Federal Trade Commission. (2007). Paying final respects: Your rights when buying funeral goods and services. https://www.ftc.gov.

Valentine, C., & Woodthorpe, K. (2014). From the cradle to the grave: Funeral welfare from an international perspective. *Social Policy and Administration*, 48(5), 515–536. https://doi.org/10.1111/spol.12018.

Waugh, E. (1948). *The loved one*. Little, Brown.

Chapter 6

Funerals and Complicated Experiences with Grief

Marlon was a longtime member of the Canadian Royal Legion in his town and his best buddies were his fellow Legionnaires with whom he gathered in the local Legion hall's bar most afternoons. There, they shot pool, had a few beers, and griped about national and provincial politics. He and Bonnie occasionally went together to Legion dinners and Bonnie participated in the women's auxiliary. Once, she even remarked to a friend, "Some people have their church, but we're not into all that religious mumbo jumbo; I guess the Legion is our church." What even a casual observer would note, however, was that Marlon and Bonnie rarely did things together, and especially since his retirement from the railroad, they had largely led "separate lives."

Even though it was widely known in their tight-knit community that Marlon and Bonnie "had problems" in their marriage, no one in town—including their adult children who lived nearby—had any inkling of how desperate life had become. Apparently, the recent financial downturn had left them scrambling with too much debt and too little income. Bonnie was known to enjoy a glass of sherry or a fine wine, but in recent years, Marlon's alcohol consumption had become more serious. Even his doctor had warned him about the amount of alcohol he was consuming and how hard that made his body work in light of his heart disease, diabetes, and poor kidney function. His drinking also had sent his weight in the wrong direction; he had added about 15 kg since his last checkup.

The provincial police received a 911 call about eleven thirty one night from an apartment on the west side. The caller said she had heard arguing coming from Marlon and Bonnie's apartment next door much of the evening, that it had intensified, and then, she heard three loud bangs—she thought they were gunshots—and then her next-door neighbor's apartment fell silent. Upon arrival, the police and paramedics confirmed what they had suspected based on the 911 caller's report. It appeared that Marlon had shot his wife in the head in a fit of rage and then shot himself in the head. Bonnie's body was across the living room on the sofa; Marlon's was lying in the hallway and his pistol lay beside

DOI: 10.4324/9781003353010-7

him. Three shell casings were on the floor, and one bullet was embedded in the wall right above Bonnie's body. Police surmised that what the caller reported was likely a missed first shot, followed by the second shot that killed Bonnie, and then a third shot with which Marlon killed himself.

Even before friends started gathering at the Legion Hall on Saturday morning, the town was abuzz with talk of what had happened. After the medical examiner released Marlon's and Bonnie's bodies, the local funeral director had them cremated at the family's request, and the Legion, with their adult children's blessing, went to work planning a "celebration of life" at the Legion Hall for the two of them. Marlon and Bonnie's eldest son said he wanted a funeral for his mom; he was not sure he would even attend one for his dad. His younger sisters and friends at the Legion, with the help of the funeral director (who was also a Legionnaire), persuaded him that Marlon's life was not defined by this one act in the end and that the family and community needed to gather to honor the "whole man," rather than focus only on the final deed of his life.

As expected, the memorial service was difficult for the family, for Marlon and Bonnie's closest friends, and for the other nearly 200 community members who gathered in the Legion Hall that Sunday afternoon, eight days after the couple had died. The officiant for the service was the Legion's chaplain who had at least had experience with these kinds of difficult funerals. He had spent his professional career as a chaplain for 25 years in the Royal Canadian Air Force, the very branch of military in which Marlon had served. The chaplain reflected on the influence that Bonnie and Marlon had on their community, their active involvement in the Legion, their care for low-income veterans in their town, and their investment in their children and grandchildren. Several people stood during the "open mic" portion of the service and paid tribute to Marlon's and Bonnie's lives. Several speakers implied that they wished they had known the depths of despair that must have characterized Marlon's life in the end.

A few days after the memorial service, the chaplain and funeral director had morning coffee together at the funeral home. Together, they agreed it had been among the most difficult services of their respective careers. Both had taken care of such funerals a few times in the past but never for a couple so well loved and with whom they were friends. The chaplain even noted that he considered it one of the most important moments of his ministry: "I got to use my gifts to help my friends begin to make sense of an experience that makes no sense. There is nothing more important that I have ever done."

Domains of Complicated Grief

With the codification of prolonged grief disorder (PGD; American Psychiatric Association, 2022) as a constellation of clinically significant bereavement symptoms that do not abate, there has been broad—though not unanimous—consensus that some grief does not seemingly get easier over time. The new term introduces into the clinical lexicon an official term for what has been variously called pathological grief (Gort, 1984; Parkes, 1965), traumatic grief (Prigerson et al., 1999), and complicated grief (Shear et al., 2005), though the clinical criteria of these terms often differ somewhat from one another. Although the criteria for the American Psychiatric Association's (2022) definition of PGD is considerably more detailed than that of the World Health Organization (2022), both note that the symptoms include such features as persistent longing for and preoccupation with the deceased, exaggerated emotional responses (rage, guilt, blame, etc.), and inability to experience pleasure following the death of a loved one. The criteria for the *Diagnostic and Statistical Manual of Mental Disorders* (DSM-5-TR; American Psychiatric Association, 2022) specify that the symptoms of this "disordered" grief have persisted for a year after the death while the *International Classification of Disease* (World Health Organization, 2022) allows a diagnosis of disorder at the six-month mark post-death.

Although there is wide consensus about the use of these terms and definitions, bereavement clinicians and scholars have certainly not spoken with one voice. Some have raised significant objection to the movement toward pathologizing human adjustment in general (Wakefield & Schmitz, 2014) and to the movement toward pathologizing complex experiences with bereavement specifically (Schuurman, 2023). Hoy (2016) posited,

> When thinking of complicated grief, much of the literature assumes that either an individual does or does not meet the condition with little "gray area" in between. This is not surprising, since for the purposes of research, a condition of study must be either present or not present; in the same way that a person is either pregnant or she is not, the research literature concerning complicated grief implies either one meets the conditions of the emerging disorder or the individual does not. As many readers . . . undoubtedly know, however, the clinical reality of complicated grief is far more complex, with levels of complication existing along a spectrum of complexity and severity.
>
> (p. 155)

In a large cross-sectional study of 1,137 respondents, Thieleman and colleagues (2023) reported that even though a significant number met the clinical criteria for PGD even several years after the loss, 98.1% of respondents indicated they did not believe their grief was abnormal or unhealthy. When asked if being told by a professional that their grief was a mental disorder would be helpful, 11.8% indicated it would be helpful and 54.9% indicated it would be very unhelpful (p. 835).

Although there are many symptom lists and schema to describe complicated grief, Hoy (2016) suggested that the elements that present risk factors for complicated grief can be divided into three somewhat overlapping domains. The *situational* domain includes the age of both the deceased and the bereaved individual as well as the circumstances surrounding the death. Deaths to young people are virtually all seen as "deaths out of time" that occur outside the "natural order" of expected life. "Parents are not supposed to bury their children" is the plaintive cry all funeral directors have heard as they met with families to plan memorial ceremonies for their newly deceased offspring. There is something deeply tragic about the death of a young mother from cancer or a young soldier killed in the line of duty.

Deaths to relatively young people not only seem "out of time," but these deaths are also often caused by traumatic injury. When a car crash, homicide, or suicide is the manner of death, surviving family members are frequently tormented by the trauma itself so that the resultant grief is often accompanied by high levels of traumatic stress. When families seek to arrange memorial ceremonies in the immediate aftermath of these kinds of death, they are often still in significant shock when creating and participating in the funeral. Worden (2018) has suggested that one feature that "dilutes" the effectiveness of funerals is when they happen too quickly after the death and family members are still "dazed or numb" (p. 121). The situation of these deaths raises the risk that grief will be harder to enfold into the bereaved person's future life.

The situational aspects of early grief are further complicated when legal requirements delay cultural or religious ceremonies. Judaism and Islam, for example, religiously prescribe that funerals be held without delay. Judaism has long held that the body should be buried intact and some rabbis have said that steps should be taken to ensure that even severed limbs and blood-soaked clothing is buried with the deceased. Rabbis have traditionally held that autopsies can be performed when necessary to satisfy legal or civil requirements (e.g., a homicide or accident investigation) but that all tissues and fluid should be returned with the body to be buried in a Jewish cemetery (Lamm, 1969; Popovsky, 2007). Even when rabbis find it permissible for a deceased person to undergo a postmortem exam, however, it is vital to remember that this may still be upsetting to the family and community, especially when such postmortem examinations delay funeral proceedings by several days.

Support is the second domain that, when absent in the experience, elevates the individual's risk for difficulties in integrating the loss. In addition to the culturally prescribed or religiously defined rituals themselves, support can be experienced by bereaved individuals in their feeling of how many and how significantly others seem emotionally present for them in their loss. The durability of faith and philosophical beliefs explored in Chapter 3 is also a measure of support, and individuals whose worldview has been shattered by this loss can also feel very alienated from an important support system.

Exploring the contours of the support system that is present in the loss is what is envisioned by Doka (2002) and others to conceptualize "disenfranchised grief." Traditionally, grief after AIDS deaths was disenfranchised, and now deaths from addiction and abuse can be added to that list. Parents whose baby died in miscarriage can feel the stinging message from society, the media, and even their own families that their child was "not really a child" and they are therefore not entitled to grieve. The grief of adults with cognitive or intellectual disabilities is often overlooked rather than being acknowledged through the making of an intentional space in memorial ceremonies for their attendance and even participation. Anytime bereaved individuals sense a lack of support in their experience with loss, they are at an elevated risk for problematic, long-term difficulties in accommodating the loss.

Culturally prescribed rituals are essential to healthy grieving for individuals who subscribe to those cultural practices, and there is documented complication in cases where, for example, a public health emergency prohibits those rituals. Chapter 7 addresses these issues in the COVID-19 global pandemic, but there are many other examples on a more local scale without widespread media attention. The West African Ebola outbreak of 2014 centered on Guinea, Liberia, and Sierra Leone raised new questions about the intersection of safe handling of decedents, culturally vital rituals, and the bereavement of families and communities.

Moran's (2017) ethnographic analysis of burial practices and health edicts during the Ebola crisis sheds light on an often-overlooked principle. For groups with highly prescribed death rituals, completion of those rituals, even in the face of personal risk, is vital not only in an esoteric spiritual sense to prevent the deceased's spirits from haunting the living, but also as a vital aspect of their own bereavement work. Moran pointed out that since young journalists have such poor understanding of rituals and bereavement in their own cultures, it comes as little surprise they would struggle to understand different cultural groups (p. 402). The mandated cremation of all corpses in Monrovia, Liberia in the fall of 2014 was an affront to local sensibilities and clearly a complicating factor in the bereavement experiences of families and communities. As an anthropologist, Moran (2017) asked rhetorically, "How differently would we interpret the rage expressed by many communities against health workers and burial teams if we situated it within frameworks of bereavement rather than a fear of 'spirits' and suspicion of Western medicine?" (p. 417).

A final domain of complicated grief is what Hoy (2016) called the *selfhood*, defined regularly in his writing and presentation as "the person who was already there before bereavement ever got here." No individual comes to loss as a "blank slate" but rather brings a plethora of healthy and unhealthy coping mechanisms as well as a varied and unique life experience that predates the loss. When an individual senses there is unfinished business or ambivalence in the relationship—as there so often is in the cases of substance addiction and abuse—the chances seem higher that this loss will require some additional support to accommodate.

When loss is complicated by a preexisting physical illness in the bereaved individual, the use of particular medications and the fatigue that may accompany that illness can significantly reduce a person's natural resilience. Chronic pain reduces ability to cope in virtually every arena of life, especially in emotional coping (Hampton et al., 2019; Malfliet et al., 2017). As one mother with fibromyalgia put it following the death of her young adult daughter, "I was already 'running on fumes' with very little reserve in 'the tank' when she died." There is long-standing awareness that even the grief after an expected death to an older person can occasion significant emotional disruption for a person with underlying depression, an anxiety disorder, or a personality disorder such as borderline personality disorder (Hoy, 2016, especially chap. 7).

Fatal Substance Overdoses

Overdoses from substances have become an epidemic across the globe with more than 600,000 deaths attributed to drug use in 2019. Opioid narcotics, which include some of the biggest killers like morphine and fentanyl, are formulated to control pain, but one of the side effects is that they also tend to suppress respiration. Although temporary suppression of respiration is not generally of concern in a controlled medical environment, the phenomenon quickly becomes fatal when too much of the drug is taken (World Health Organization, 2023a).

In a cross-sectional study of 1,137 bereaved respondents, Thieleman and colleagues (2023) found that the highest prevalence of complicated grief (meeting the DSM-5-TR criteria for PGD) were survivors whose loved one had died of a substance overdose with 59.1% of respondents meeting the criteria for PGD. Although the average time since the loss was 10.16 years, rate of PGD remained above 35% until reaching the ten-year mark. For those bereaved from one to two years, 53.9% met the criteria (p. 834).

Bereaved family members and friends are at an elevated risk of complicated grief responses after a loved one dies from a drug overdose. Feigelman and colleagues (2011) found no significant differences in bereavement responses between parents whose child died from suicide or from a drug overdose but found the grief was significantly more troubling for those parents than for the second subgroup, those whose children had died from accidents and natural causes. Of 575 bereaved parents in their sample, 80% of the parents reported their son or daughter was between the ages of 16 and 35 at death. A total of 48 reported their child died from accidental drug overdose.

Feigelman and colleagues (2011, p. 303) asked several open-ended questions about the role of stigma in grief and tabulated a total of 2,421 responses, 1,541 of which were negative responses about being stigmatized or feeling stigmatized as a result of their child's death. Their results indicated that parents of children who died by drug overdose endure much of the same stigmatization and exclusionary behavior as those whose children died from suicide. Reported grief difficulties, post-traumatic stress, complicated grief, depression, and psychological problems were similar between parents whose children died by suicide and those who died by drug overdose, but these reports were considerably more prevalent than among both of these groups than among those whose children died from accidents or natural causes.

Among this group of parents, there were significant numbers of parents who experienced the failure of empathy on the part of associates and family members. Some of these others blamed the child, with one stating the child "was better off dead because he was already doomed from his lifelong mental illness or drug addiction" (p. 312). Other parents experienced blame aimed at them as a parent for failing to act, which understandably in turn led to a heightening of self-blame. Nearly half of parents experienced blaming responses from one or more persons significant to them. "These experiences help to sustain a mood of shame, reticence, and extreme caution for these bereaved in their interactions with non-survivors" (p. 312).

Funerals in such a setting as this are particularly difficult. Upon realizing the likelihood that parents might be blaming themselves and that community mourners might be blaming either the parents or the deceased, one clergyperson acknowledged that fact in the funeral with words like, "You know, the research says that it is common for us to blame ourselves or to blame each other in a time like this. We wonder what did you or I miss? What could have been different? Those are valid questions we won't likely get answered in this life. But we can learn to trust God and share His grace with one another. That is what I would like to talk about here today."

Traumatic Accidents and Memorial Ceremonies

The shock that accompanies traumatic death makes memorialization in these contexts particularly challenging. Not only does family and community face an unexpected death, but also there is often substantial damage to the body. Families who may most need to "see to believe" can be stymied in their efforts because the corpse is not regarded as "viewable" by others, including health-care and law enforcement professionals (Hoy, 2023). In their grounded theory–influenced qualitative study of 16 individuals bereaved after sudden death, Harrington and Sprowl (2011) noted that "participants that were denied an early viewing repeatedly described a persistent feeling that something was missing, a void or remaining emptiness" (p. 78).

Giannopoulou and colleagues (2021) found among 168 adolescents exposed to a single mass casualty bus accident in which seven peers were killed that many survivors exhibited high symptoms of post-traumatic stress disorder (PTSD) and persistent grief over time. More than one-fifth of the students exhibited high and unremitting levels of grief over time. Although more than one-fifth of students had significantly resolved issues related to problematic grief by 18 months post-loss, there remained a significant danger for clinically significant symptoms to persist. The researchers found no correlation between having been on the scene (witnessed rather than viewing on news coverage) and higher levels of persistent grief. There was no discussion in the research study of funeral or memorial rituals in which the peers may have participated, though there was evidence that higher levels of social support at 18 months post-loss was associated with better overall functioning. The researchers posited that social support is difficult to achieve and measure in a small community where so many people are impacted by the same incident. Although there is likely solidarity in shared loss, the shared loss itself may complicate the actual provision and reception of support.

In a sweeping study of Balinese family survivors of individuals killed in car crashes, Djelantik and colleagues (2021) surveyed and interviewed 301 participants from 103 families a mean of 16 months after a fatal motor vehicle crash. Participants were 95% Hindu, and all but one respondent participated in culturally prescribed funeral rituals following the death. Depression scores for the majority of respondents (79%) demonstrated no measurable level of depression while 19% scored within the range for "mild depression." No respondents scored above the cut-off point for PGD, while four respondents (1%) scored above the cut-off point for PTSD (p. 776).

In discussing their results, the researchers posit that faith and beliefs, coupled with the role of funeral rituals and the social support they engender, might account for the unusually low rates of depression, PTSD, and PGD in this population. They conclude, "Certain aspects of Balinese culture protect bereaved individuals from developing mental health problems; that finding might be used to refine bereavement rituals in other cultures and perspectives on treatment of PGD" (Djelantik et al., 2021, p. 779).

In a fascinating ethnographic case study, Grønseth (2018) reported on the rituals and aftermath of a Sri Lankan Tamil refugee killed in an industrial accident in a coastal Norwegian fish processing plant. Although there was no Hindu priest to officiate at the ritual and no facility in which to complete a traditional cremation, the Catholic and Protestant clergy of the community worked together to help the family create a meaningful ceremony to honor their loved one. In planning the funeral, family and friends were concerned that the service would not seem "too exotic" to their Norwegian neighbors, creating a "greater gap between Tamils and Norwegians," said one longtime friend of the deceased. "The gap will be filled with racism. We do not want that" (p. 2622).

As planned, on the day of the funeral, mourners assembled at the site of the accident and joined in the funeral procession to the community's Protestant church that had offered to host the ceremony. Family and friends, many of them wearing garlands, walked behind the hearse carrying the deceased's open casket through the town streets as dozens of Norwegians looked on. While the Norwegians did not join in the pedestrian procession, they did drive to the church for the service. A Catholic priest, himself of Tamil ethnicity serving in Oslo, played Tamil-Hindu songs from a tape player and included Vedic and Sanskrit texts in the funeral ceremony.

The *tali* is a necklace-type symbol Tamil wives wear from their wedding until their husband's death. Under normal circumstances, the Tamil wife would throw her *tali* onto her husband's funeral pyre, but since there was no cremation to be done in this Norwegian town, she instead threw the ornament into her husband's coffin in a moment of deep mourning witnessed by all. After the funeral had ended, the coffin was shipped to Sri Lanka for cremation and his employer paid the expenses.

Grønseth (2018) went on to explain that many of the Tamil in the community feared the ghost of the deceased. He had died in a tragic accident, which might cause his ghost to wander, they thought. Moreover, the cremation of his body was delayed for some time and that could cause the ghost to be restless as well. While family and friends had venerated his picture and offered food and drink in his home, the hope was that his ghost was satisfied, but few seemed sure.

The funeral, Grønseth (2018) suggested, had demonstrated the Tamil's unique ways of attempting to "fit into" their new culture while not completely relinquishing the ways of their old one. "Thus, I suggest that the funeral is a 'double rite of passage:' not only Bala's (the deceased) passage from life to death, but also a possible passage for Tamils generally from not-belonging to [the becoming of] belonging" (pp. 2626–2627).

Certainly, some native Norwegians also were saddened by the death of the young Tamil refugee worker. Their choices to participate in the funeral no doubt demonstrated solidarity with the grieving refugee family and community, allowing the unique funeral ritual to provide a healing balm for a hurting town.

For many reasons, it seems accidental deaths occur more frequently among young people, which causes significant upheaval among parents, peers, and the community at large. Many cases of multiple fatalities in a single automobile crash involve the young, and these funerals—whether a single fatality or multiple fatality—represent difficulties in the death-related ceremonies.

First, traumatic injuries to the body are more often present with accidental deaths, which forces family and friends to confront the real/not-real questions surrounding the death. Well-meaning professionals may try to protect parents from seeing their recently deceased teen or young adult children, an issue clarified in interviews and reported by Harrington and Sprowl (2011).

Second, accidental deaths—and all deaths by traumatic circumstances—raise questions about life's meaning. The world is suddenly seen as unpredictable and capricious, especially for peers of the deceased who may have previously sensed some level of invincibility. By involving peers of the deceased in funeral ceremonies, they will more likely begin the process of creating meaning. In the same way that kinesthetic activities tend to improve learning outcomes, it is likely that active involvement in funeral ceremonies help anchor peers' memories to the place and emotional meanings of the funeral, thereby potentially contributing to better grief outcomes.

Funerals after Suicide

Arguably the most important historical voice in suicidology, Edwin Shneidman (1969) wrote that the person dying by suicide "puts his psychological skeleton in the survivor's emotional closet. He sentences the survivor to a complex of negative feelings and, most importantly, to obsess about the reasons for the death" (p. 22). Reflecting on four decades of working therapeutically with suicide survivors, Jordan (2020) noted that there has been wide-ranging acceptance in research and clinical literature suggesting that suicide bereavement is different from other types of loss in that there tends to be a greater sense of guilt among survivors, more intense levels of shame and stigmatization, and a greater sense of social isolation in the aftermath of the death. His observation, however, is that it is the "perceived intentionality" on the part of the deceased that most characterizes this loss (p. 2). He observes further that the mystery surrounding the deceased's intent is baffling to survivors and their community as people muse, "Of course, everyone wants to keep living, don't they?" (p. 3).

Globally, more than 700,000 individuals die annually from suicide with an outsized portion of those deaths in under-resourced countries. More than 20% of global suicides occur through pesticide self-poisoning, and this manner of death is particularly prevalent in low-income countries (World Health Organization, 2023b). After many years of declines, suicide rates in the United States, like some other countries, appear to have risen in recent years. Although the data are far from conclusive, the global COVID-19 pandemic and its aftermath addressed in Chapter 7 likely exacerbated the growing number of individuals who contemplate, attempt, and complete self-harm (Pathirathna et al., 2022). The emotional fallout for families and for entire communities can be far reaching following a death from suicide.

Known risk factors for suicide include a history of mental disorders such as depression, alcohol use disorders, and a previous suicide attempt. Nevertheless, many of these deaths occur in moments of impulsivity related to a crisis or an inability to deal with stresses such as financial reversal, relational breakups, interpersonal violence, and chronic pain or illness (World Health Organization, 2023b).

Sometimes one or more of these "assumed causes" is well known to family and even to the wider community when the death occurs, leading many families to name or at least to speculate on the circumstances that led to the death. This behavior can be part of the process of creating meaning of an otherwise-unexplainable event but can also become the means for blaming an individual or group. One clergyperson recounted a particularly uncomfortable moment when, at the visitation of an adolescent girl, the boyfriend who had broken up with her the day before her death showed up. From across the room, this minister recalled, the girl's mother yelled, "Get that f**king murderer out of my sight!"

Memorial ceremonies after suicides range from disarmingly honest accounts of the circumstances leading to the death to services with no mention whatsoever of the death's circumstances. In interviews, funeral directors report the increasing likelihood that families are forthright in the funeral ceremonies and even in published obituary notices. One funeral director pointed to a statement written by a family on her own website to demonstrate how some families publicize the facts (names and identifying details are redacted to protect the family's anonymity). In the obituary statement, after describing several difficult life experiences through which the deceased had recently walked, the family wrote, "In the stress of this environment and against a backdrop of a years-long struggle with depression, he could no longer face the world. That collided with an overwhelming urge to end the pain and he took his life."

In interviews, clergy consistently say that funeral ceremonies for individuals who have died by suicide are often the most difficult they face, a concept echoed by Roberts (2017) when he wrote to colleagues in the clergy, "The most difficult funeral of all will be when a person has ended her/his own life. No experience in your repertoire is equivalent to dealing with a death through suicide" (p. 12). Preparing remarks in such settings is especially difficult because some family members may be very comfortable with disclosing the details while others expect to keep those details hidden. Even though legally, one person usually gets to decide, one minister noted, it is "vital to walk a line that ministers to everyone present if at all possible."

An experienced funeral celebrant reported the memorial ceremonies for a man who had immolated himself in his own car as a suicide means. At the end of the funeral, several family members were insistent on seeing his body one last time, and the celebrant reported his own discomfort at remaining close at hand to support the adult siblings of the man as they viewed his badly disfigured body. This suicide was particularly complex, according to the officiant, because the "manifesto" the deceased had written indicated he was sacrificing himself in a government protest and he completed his act in front of a government building. His family assumed from his letter that he intended his act not only to end his own life but also to destroy the building.

Jordan (2020) noted several psychological tasks needed by suicide survivors to fully integrate their loss, including "containment of the trauma with a restoration of psychological safety, . . . repair of the mourner's assumptive world, . . . [and] repair of the relationship with the deceased" (pp. 3–5). One task that is especially salient for funerals, however, is Jordan's task of "development of a durable biography of the deceased," which he noted typically begins at the funeral and likely continues for years.

Caregivers can likely help ensure these tasks are begun by acknowledging the questions that arise for mourners while also leading families and communities to think about the person's death in the fuller context of an entire life. Often, family members describe admirable character qualities and behaviors: "He would have given you the shirt off his back" or "She worked hard to make sure everyone was included" or "If he had one dollar left, he would give it to somebody in need." One experienced funeral celebrant recounted echoing the exact words heard in his interview with family members in his remarks in the service by saying, "Jackie recalls her brother was a man of incredible generosity and gratitude." Jordan (2020) noted that this aspect of remembering might be among the most difficult with individuals bereaved by a loved one's suicide death because the focus can become about the death itself rather than the stories that "predate" the death (p. 6), a phenomenon illustrated in the case of Marlon and Bonnie that opened this chapter.

Homicide and the Difficulties of Memorials

Although not as prevalent as deaths by suicide, homicide ends the lives of more than 460,000 people globally each year. Defined in the United Nations Office on Drugs and Crime (2019) International Classification of Crime for Statistical Purposes, homicide is the "unlawful death inflicted upon a person with the intent to cause death or serious injury" (p. 9). In the introduction to its report on homicide, the United Nations report noted, "Intentional homicide is the ultimate crime and has ripple effects that go far beyond the original loss of human life. For homicide also blights the lives of the victim's family and community, who may therefore be described as 'secondary victims.' It creates a violent environment that has a negative impact on society, the economy and government institutions" (p. 9).

Schaal and colleagues (2010) found among the 400 participants of their study that genocide had a deleterious and long-lasting impact on the bereavement experience of survivors. More than 8% of their Rwandan widows and orphans met the criteria that would eventually be defined as PGD, even though respondents were an average of 12 years post-loss. Expectedly, among widows and orphans whose loved ones had died in the 1994 Rwandan genocide, the prevalence of PGD was demonstrably higher. Research participants who reported their loved one's death was violent, who experienced high levels of PTSD symptoms, whose grief related to a recent loss, and who reported no importance to religious/spiritual beliefs were the participants who were most likely to exhibit high levels of grief.

In a grounded theory study of 37 surviving family members of the 1995 massacre of 4,000 men in Srebrenica, Bosnia-Herzegovina, Pollack (2003) found differences between survivors who were involved in political advocacy versus those who were not. When bones were recovered several years after the massacre and government officials determined to bury them in a communal memorial, those who were uninvolved in political advocacy groups saw the burial as a primary tool in facilitating family and communal mourning. For those who were involved in political advocacy, the meaning ascribed to the burial of the remains was acknowledgment of the genocide and the bloodshed that was the cost for the birth of a new state. Moreover, Pollack found that among Bosnian Muslim informants, there was deep relief that their loved ones could finally rest. In their commonly held belief, spirits tended to wander aimlessly and restlessly until the body was appropriately prepared and buried.

Rival's (2005) riveting ethnographic study of the Amazonian Huarorani found that the most honorable death among this people group is to be speared (murdered) by another and that this type of death is far more honorable than to die in old age. Anthropologists have reported cases where warriors were buried with a child so that they would not be destined to leave their "homeland" alone. Although codified into the burial customs of the Huarorani, these customs may not be that unlike Westerners who create "heroic honors" for fallen soldiers, firefighters, and police officers. These heroes seem to be accorded "double honor" when their death was in sacrifice for another such as is the case for a soldier killed when he falls on a grenade to preserve the life of his squad.

Clinical Implications

Whether an individual meets the criteria for PGD and regardless of whether the clinician believes such a taxonomy should even exist, that individual whose experience with loss is complicated by any of the factors explored in this chapter presents a unique challenge to the counselor or support group leader who provides care. In the immediate aftermath of a death in traumatic or unexpected circumstances, providers can suggest to family members (and the larger community) the importance of slowing down. Although the luxury of time was often not afforded in the height of the COVID-19 pandemic, under normal circumstances there is no compelling reason not to take some time.

In instructions to caregivers for arranging funerals after a traumatic death, professionals and supportive volunteers are urged to pay special attention to the role of shock that could delay processing and therefore effectiveness of the memorial ceremonies. Moreover, caregivers must be alert to the availability of the body and its condition for viewing if that is part of the family's tradition since unexpected deaths and unmet expectations can further complicate the loss. Care providers must attend to the possibility there is disenfranchisement from a supportive community or from a previously held set of core beliefs, and we are prudent to investigate how the bereaved individual's perception of these additional losses might complicate grief. Whether arranging funerals after traumatic circumstances or reflecting with bereaved individuals about them later, caregivers are wise to inquire about how the events of the death fit into the total picture of life. Often, resetting the manner of death into the context of life's core values and character qualities is a vital part of bereavement support and counseling, and the astute counselor can simply ask, "In what ways was the way your brother died *not* like the way he lived his life?" (Hoy, 2023).

When a person dies after an extended or chronic illness in advanced age, one is tempted to see the cause of death as the period at the end of the sentence. However, when a death comes by accident, homicide, or suicide, the punctuation mark at the end of the sentence is an exclamation point or a question mark. In many profound ways, the cause and manner of death is the very important punctuation mark in the sentence. In grammar, a sentence's punctuation is vital for the reader because it indicates inflection and emphasis, but it is not the whole sentence. Rather, the nouns, verbs, adjectives, and adverbs make up the heart of the message getting communicated.

In a similar vein, knowing the cause of death is important for good clinical work in bereavement to occur, but it is not the whole story—in bereavement counseling or in the recasting of the biographical narrative of the person who died. Rather, one of the most important aspects of supportive work with grieving people is to help them re-create a new biography that certainly does not exclude the cause and manner of death but rather incorporates those facts as part of the entire story of this person's life and legacy.

Asking during the counseling conversation, "How did the funeral or memorial ceremony start you on the process of creating a new biography or story of your sister's life?" can be an important diagnostic question. In all likelihood, the bereaved individual has not thought about the creation of a new life story that includes—but does not highlight only—the cause and manner of death. Many helpers err on one side or the other, either completely ignoring the circumstances of the death or talking about nothing else in an attempt to address any underlying trauma.

An additional direction for a counseling conversation is to inquire about how the bereaved wishes the rituals would have been different, or in the case there were not any, what the individual would have included in the ceremony. In cases where there has been no ceremony after a traumatic death, I have worked with bereaved individuals to create an entire ritual, deciding what music would be shared, what the eulogy would include, and what photos would be displayed. I have listened to playlists with bereaved individuals, leafed through photo albums with them, and listened as they read heartfelt eulogies aloud.

In one case, a bereaved mom whose son had been cremated without any service felt unable to read aloud the eulogy she had written between our meetings. She had worked on the document over several weeks and finally passed it over to me during our conversation, asking me if I would read it aloud. As I began reading the words she had written out of her heartbroken spirit, something amazing happened in that clinical encounter. I read her own words back to her, and she heard them aloud in an emotionally safe space while I simply "bore witness" to both her pain and her son's legacy that her words recorded. In a profound way, she held a funeral in my consultation room that afternoon, and even though they were her words, having them uttered aloud seemed to seal it in her memory much more than simply rehearsing those characteristics in her own mind and heart (Hoy, 2023, p. 54).

Reflection and Discussion

- What is the "hardest" funeral or memorial service in which you have participated or attended? What made it particularly difficult?
- How do you think the author's "domains of complicated grief"—situation, support, and selfhood—relate to the role of memorial ceremonies? Which domain do you think would create the most challenges in ceremonies?

- What specifically could you do to increase support to individuals whose loved one has died in complicated circumstances? What might the role of stigma, shame, blame, or anger be?

References

American Psychiatric Association. (2022). *Diagnostic and statistical manual of mental disorders* (5th ed., text rev.). American Psychiatric Association.

Djelantik, A.A.A.M.J., Aryani, P., Boelen, P.A., Lesmana, C.B.J., & Kleber, R.J. (2021). Prolonged grief disorder, posttraumatic stress disorder, and depression following traffic accidents among bereaved Balinese family members: Prevalence, latent classes and cultural correlates. *Journal of Affective Disorders, 292*, 773–781. https://doi.org/10.1016/j.jad.2021.05.085.

Doka, K.J. (Ed.). (2002). *Disenfranchised grief: New directions, challenges, and strategies for practice*. Research Press.

Feigelman, W., Jordan, J.R., & Gorman, B.S. (2011). Parental grief after a child's drug death compared to other death causes: Investigating a greatly neglected bereavement population. *Omega: Journal of Death and Dying*, 63(4), 291–316. https://doi.org/10.2190/OM.63.4.a.

Giannopoulou, I., Richardson, C., & Papadatou, D. (2021). Peer loss: Posttraumatic stress, depression, and grief symptoms in a traumatized adolescent community. *Clinical Child Psychology and Psychiatry*, 26(2), 556–568. https://doi.org/10.1177/1359104520980028.

Gort, G. (1984). Pathological grief: Causes, recognition, and treatment. *Canadian Family Physician (Medecin de Famille Canadien)*, 30, 914–924.

Grønseth, A.S. (2018). Migrating rituals: Negotiations of belonging and otherness among Tamils in Norway. *Journal of Ethnic and Migration Studies*, 44(16), 2617–2633. https://doi.org/10.1080/1369183X.2017.1389026.

Hampton, S.N., Nakonezny, P.A., Richard, H.M., & Wells, J.E. (2019). Pain catastrophizing, anxiety, and depression in hip pathology. *The Bone & Joint Journal, 101-B*(7), 800–807. https://doi.org/10.1302/0301-620X.101B7.BJJ-2018-1309.R1.

Harrington, C., & Sprowl, B. (2011). Family members' experiences with viewing in the wake of sudden death. *Omega: Journal of Death and Dying*, 64(1), 65–82. https://doi.org/10.2190/OM.64.1.e.

Hoy, W.G. (2016). *Bereavement groups and the role of social support: Integrating theory, research, and practice*. Routledge.

Hoy, W.G. (2023). Funerals and memorialization after trauma. In D.A. Balk, T. Wong, & J.D. Balk (Eds.), *A professional's guide to understanding trauma and loss* (chap.14). Cambridge Scholars Press.

Jordan, J.R. (2020). Lessons learned: Forty years of clinical work with suicide loss survivors. *Frontiers in Psychology*, 11, 766–766. https://doi.org/10.3389/fpsyg.2020.00766.

Lamm, M. (1969). *The Jewish way in death and mourning*. Jonathan David Publishers.

Malfliet, A., Coppieters, I., Van Wilgen, P., Kregel, J., De Pauw, R., Dolphens, M., & Ickmans, K. (2017). Brain changes associated with cognitive and emotional factors in chronic pain: A systematic review. *European Journal of Pain*, 21(5), 769–786. https://doi.org/10.1002/ejp.1003.

Moran, M.H. (2017). Missing bodies and secret funerals: The production of "safe and dignified burials" in the Liberian Ebola crisis. *Anthropological Quarterly*, 90(2), 399–421. https://doi.org/10.1353/anq.2017.0024.

Parkes, C.M. (1965). Bereavement and mental illness: A clinical study of the grief of bereaved psychiatric patients. *British Journal of Medical Psychology*, 38(3), 1–12. https://doi.org/10.1111/j.2044-8341.1965.tb00956.x.

Pathirathna, M.L., Nandasena, H.M.R.K.G., Atapattu, A.M.M.P., & Weeraskara, I. (2022). Impact of the COVID-19 pandemic on suicidal attempts and death rates: A systematic review. *BMC Psychiatry, 22*(506), 1–15. https://doi.org/10.1186/s12888-022-04158-w.

Pollack, C.E. (2003). Intentions of burial: Mourning, politics, and memorials following the massacre at Srebrenica. *Death Studies*, 27(2), 125–142. https://doi.org/10.1080/07481180302893.

Popovsky, M.A. (2007, May). *Jewish ritual, reality, and response at the end of life: A guide to caring for Jewish patients and their families*. Duke Institute on Care at the End of Life/Duke Divinity School. https://www.iceol.duke.edu.

Prigerson, H.G., Shear, M.K., Jacobs, S.C., Reynolds, C.F., 3rd, Maciejewski, P.K., Davidson, J.R., Rosenheck, R., Pilkonis, P.A., Wortman, C.B., Williams, J.B., Widiger, T.A., Frank, E., Kupfer, D.J., & Zisook, S. (1999). Consensus criteria for traumatic grief: A preliminary empirical test. *The British Journal of Psychiatry*, 174, 67–73. https://doi.org/10.1192/bjp.174.1.67.

Rival, L. (2005). The attachment of the soul to the body among the Huaorani of Amazonian Ecuador. *Ethnos*, 70(3), 285–310. https://doi.org/10.1080/00141840500294300.

Roberts, D.A. (2017). Preparing a eulogy or memorial service for one who died by suicide. In M. Moore & D.A. Roberts (Eds.), *The suicide funeral (or memorial service): Honoring their memory, comforting their survivors* (pp.54–63). Resource Publications.

Schaal, S., Jacob, N., Dusingizemungu, J.-P., & Elbert, T. (2010). Rates and risks for prolonged grief disorder in a sample of orphaned and widowed genocide survivors. *BMC Psychiatry*, 10(1), 55–55. https://doi.org/10.1186/1471-244X-10-55.

Schuurman, D.L. (2023, April 27). *Flawed foundations: Deconstructing three contemporary grief constructs*. Paper presented at the Association for Death Education & Counseling, Columbus, OH.

Shear, K., Frank, E., Houck, P.R., & Reynolds, C.F., 3rd. (2005). Treatment of complicated grief: A randomized controlled trial. *Journal of the American Medical Association*, 293(21), 2601–2608. https://doi.org/10.1001/jama.293.21.2601.

Shneidman, E.S. (1969). *On the nature of suicide*. Jossey-Bass.

Streeter, R. (1831). A sermon delivered at the funeral of Miss Abigail Reed of Westford, Mass., aged twenty years: who departed this life on the tenth of September 1831, the victim of modern revivals. Spooner and Church, printers. https://link-gale-com.CY0108010460/SABN?

Thieleman, K., Cacciatore, J., & Frances, A. (2023). Rates of prolonged grief disorder: Considering relationship to the person who died and cause of death. *Journal of Affective Disorders*, 339, 832–837. https://doi.org/10.1016/j.jad.2023.07.094.

United Nations Office on Drugs and Crime. (2019). International classification of crime for statistical purposes. https://www.unodc.org.

Wakefield, J.C., & Schmitz, M.F. (2014). Uncomplicated depression, suicide attempt, and the DSM-5 bereavement exclusion debate: An empirical evaluation. *Research on Social Work Practice*, 24(1), 37–49. https://doi.org/10.1177/1049731513495092.

Worden, J.W. (2018). *Grief counseling and grief therapy: A handbook for the mental health practitioner* (5th ed.). Springer.

World Health Organization. (2022). 6B42 Prolonged grief disorder. *International classification of diseases (ICD-11) for mortality and morbidity statistics*. https://icd.who.int/browse11/l-m/en#/http://id.who.int/icd/entity/1183832314.

World Health Organization. (2023a). Opioid overdose. https://www.who/int/news-room/fact-sheets/detail/opioid-overdose.

World Health Organization. (2023b). Suicide. https://www.who.int/news-room/fact-sheets/detail/suicide.

Chapter 7

The Pandemic that Changed Everything . . . Including Funerals

After Marjorie's dad died, she had always promised her mother, "I'll be there with you to the end your life." When her mom became increasingly frail in the second decade after Marjorie's father's death, she suggested they both sell their homes and move in together into a new condominium development for people older than 55. Marjorie figured that starting their new life together in a "neutral location" might help mother and daughter work through any ensuing conflict. For four years, the two of them lived well together, traveled together, and attended the church where Marjorie's father's funeral had been held 14 years earlier.

On February 24, 2020, Marjorie received a panicked call from her mother in the early afternoon. "I know I wasn't supposed to," the breathless older woman told her on the phone, "but I was on a stool getting something from a high shelf and I fell. I'm so glad my phone was in my pocket," she explained, "because I can't seem to get up." Marjorie called a neighbor to go to her mother's aid while she drove the 20 minutes from her office. When she arrived, paramedics were already at her home. They were stabilizing her mother's badly fractured leg and the lead paramedic told Marjorie he strongly suspected she had fractured her hip in the fall. They were transporting her to a local hospital.

Marjorie's mom underwent surgery the next morning to repair her hip. Even though her initial recovery went well in light of the patient's advanced age and the other cuts and bruises she sustained in the fall, the trauma orthopedic team recommended she go to rehab for a few weeks while she healed. But just three weeks later, the governor declared all skilled nursing facilities off-limits to family visits.

The older woman asked repeatedly where her daughter was as she became increasingly agitated, confused, and withdrawn. Her hearing and sight impairments made communication with Marjorie all but impossible through phone or video chat, and the staff was so overworked that rarely did anyone have time to get the two together on a video chat anyway. Three weeks later on April 6, the nursing home called Marjorie, herself "locked down" by the governor's stay-at-home orders, to say that they

DOI: 10.4324/9781003353010-8

found her mother unresponsive and could not resuscitate her. Marjorie believes they made little effort.

However, in hearing Marjorie's story, one realizes that her mother's death "all alone and locked away from the people who cared for her" was just the beginning of the indignity. Indoor funerals in a funeral chapel or church were strictly against the law with stiff fines promised to families, congregations, or funeral directors who violated the orders. The restrictions adopted by the cemetery where Marjorie's father was buried and where her mother was also to be interred allowed for a funeral director, an officiant such as a priest or minister, and one family member to be in attendance. No one else would be allowed through the gate into the cemetery, Marjorie was told by the funeral director. Marjorie developed a nasty cough a few days before the burial was scheduled, so she was unable to attend in person; rescheduling the service would mean a delay of no less than four more weeks.

Telling her story three years later, Marjorie still reels from the devastation of the experience. She can hardly get the words out between the sobs. She has difficulty focusing at work and recognizes how angry she has become. "I promised my mom I would take care of her to the end," Marjorie plaintively explained. "Not only did she die alone, but we didn't even have a decent funeral for her."

Marjorie's story is far from unique. Millions of times in the global COVID-19 pandemic her story was repeated as families were unable to say goodbye to their loved ones or, if they were, often after the patient lost consciousness. As the world moved from fear to policy in an attempt to control an untamable virus, funerals were deeply curtailed or forbidden altogether, and mourners were sentenced to cope with their grief in seclusion and isolation without so much as a hug from caring friends and family members (Boholano & Bacus, 2022; Júnior et al., 2020; Martyr, 2023; Mas'amah et al., 2023; Testoni et al., 2021).

History of a Pandemic: From Outbreak to Shutdowns

In December 2019, a cluster of patients in Wuhan, China began experiencing symptoms of an atypical respiratory illness that proved resistant to standard treatments. By January 19, the novel coronavirus (as it became called) had been identified in laboratory tests in China, Thailand, Japan, and Korea, and a day later, the U.S. Center for Disease Control and Prevention (CDC) identified the first case in the United States. By the end of January, the World Health Organization had named the 2019 novel coronavirus a Public Health Emergency of International Concern and the U.S. Department of Health and Human Services declared it a public health emergency (U.S. Center for Disease Control and Prevention, 2023).

On February 11, the World Health Organization officially identified the new disease as COVID-19, an abbreviation of coronavirus disease 2019, and the global death toll reached 1,013 just two months after identification of the first case. Italy's nationwide Decree-Law number 6 effectively locked down that country as the nation became a COVID hotspot. Meanwhile the CDC's Nancy Messonnier held a briefing telling people to prepare for widespread school closings, canceling of public gatherings, workplace shutdowns, and other efforts to mitigate the spread of the disease, warning, "disruption to everyday life may be severe" (U.S. Center for Disease Control and Prevention, 2023, n.p.). In retrospect, these words proved prophetic though no one could appreciate how deep and wide those restrictions would become.

By mid-March, the World Health Organization labeled COVID-19 as a global pandemic, and the CDC discovered guidelines being circulated among state health departments that prioritized care for who would get respiratory ventilators in the event there was a shortage. Massachusetts and Pennsylvania used a point system to prioritize patients who were most likely to benefit from intensive care. A reactivated New York plan from 2015 utilized "exclusion criteria," a list of medical conditions making a patient ineligible for intensive care including traumatic brain injury, severe burns, or cardiac arrest. Alabama's exclusion criteria list included both "severe or profound mental retardation" and "moderate to severe dementia" (U.S. Center for Disease Control and Prevention, 2023, n.p.). By March 28, the U.S. Department of Health and Human Services (2023) responded with a civil rights bulletin of its own, reminding all health-care entities that they could not discriminate in the provision of health-care services on the basis of disability of any kind. The bulletin quoted Office of Civil Rights director Roger Severnio:

> HHS is committed to leaving no one behind during an emergency, and this guidance is designed to help health care providers meet that goal. Persons with disabilities, with limited English skills, or needing religious accommodations should not be put at the end of the line for health services during emergencies. Our civil rights laws protect the equal dignity of every human life from ruthless utilitarianism.
>
> (p. 1)

From the earliest weeks of the pandemic, emerging evidence suggested the importance of isolating individuals who had tested positive and especially those who were actively symptomatic. Virtually no one questioned the importance of protecting health-care workers using personal protective equipment (PPE), though the use of masks and face shields clearly create communication barriers, especially among those with hearing loss and those for whom the language being spoken by health-care professionals is not their first language.

Restrictions were added in different jurisdictions to "keep the public safe" with some governments taking drastic measures to separate individuals and prohibit any kind of gathering. School students were sent home to learn online, restaurants and bars closed, and all but the most basic services (sometimes called "essential services") were required under threat of fines and imprisonment to remain closed. Individuals were instructed to remain physically distant by making sure one was no closer than six feet from a non-immediate family member. Grocery stores limited the number of shoppers allowed in at any one time and lines formed quickly as people "kept their distance."

Early in the pandemic, data indicated that African American and Hispanic populations were at a higher risk of dying from COVID-19 than white populations, providing new evidence to the growing awareness of racial disparities about health care in the United States. In one report, mortality among Blacks in Chicago was six times that for whites in data from the Chicago Department of Public Health and the Cook County Medical Examiner's Office (Reyes et al., 2020). While relative numbers may be different, these health-care disparities have persisted through the end of the COVID-19 emergency.

Feyman and colleagues (2023) examined excess mortality from March to December 2020 for U.S. veterans and found that non-Hispanic white veterans experienced the smallest relative increase in mortality while Native American veterans had the highest increase. They also found that Black and Hispanic veterans had lower excess mortality than Native Americans, but excess mortality was at levels significantly higher than for non-Hispanic white veterans. They also found disparities among veterans to be lower than those reported in the general population (p. 646). Similarly, Kobo et al. (2023) found that what had been a decades-long improvement in cardiovascular mortality trends in the United States was reversed during the first year of the COVID-19 pandemic. These increases were most pronounced among Black and Hispanic adults.

The United Kingdom saw similar levels of disparities during the COVID-19 pandemic to those observed in the United States. Nafilyan and colleagues (2021) analyzed the health records of 29 million British householders to find that the age-stratified mortality rate (AMSR) during the first wave of the pandemic (January 21–August 31, 2020) among British white males was 119.1, while among health system recipients of Black African descent, the rate was 402.5. Disparities were significantly lower during the second wave of the pandemic (September 1–December 28, 2020) for most ethnic groups. However, during the second wave, the AMSR among British white males was 77.8, while for health system recipients of Bangladeshi descent, the rate was 318.7 (p. 613). Clearly, health disparities remain a problem with global reach.

Just more than three years after first declaring the existence of the pandemic and while acknowledging the novel coronavirus is a permanent element of the global health landscape, the international emergency committee managing the World Health Organization's response to the pandemic declared, "It is time to transition to long-term management of the COVID-19 pandemic . . . and that COVID-19 is now an established and ongoing health issue which no longer constitutes a public health emergency of international concern" (World Health Organization, 2023, para. 1–2).

Although the numbers were staggering and the impact of the pandemic on underserved populations around the globe was enormous, the individual human costs of deaths, economic losses, and mental health consequences of the COVID-19 pandemic can be easily lost in the focus on large numbers. Selman and colleagues (2020) noted that the absence of advance care planning and the difficulty creating such plans in emergencies, coupled with the loss of communication between dying patients and their families contributed to what would be significant challenges for bereaved individuals. Moreover, they noted, because COVID-19 increased respiratory distress, many families who were allowed to visit their loved ones in the acute dying phase witnessed labored breathing, further contributing to survivor experiences of post-traumatic stress. These complications of the grief process are explored more fully in Chapter 6.

These unusual phenomena not only created bereavement complications for survivors, Selman and colleagues (2020) noted; these same experiences also increased levels of moral distress for health-care professionals with nurses and physicians expressing extreme helplessness and a sense of failure. During the height of the pandemic, one funeral director epitomized this moral distress as he described the semi-trailer in the parking lot of his funeral home already filled as an overflow morgue, noting what many of his colleagues were undoubtedly thinking: "Everything in my training tells me to say yes, and right now, all I seem to be able to say is no." Recent studies have indicated that widespread resignations of funeral home staff, health-care workers, and especially nurses are at least in part due to these and other stresses growing out of the COVID-19 pandemic (Jarden et al., 2023).

Caring for the Dead in the Pandemic

Almost certainly, photos of bodies being "stacked like cordwood" in New York City have created unerasable images in the memories of any who saw them. The city's death-care system, like its health-care system, was overwhelmed in the early months of the pandemic with New York City's death count for March and April 2020 ringing in at 27,000, six times the pre-pandemic normal level for those two months (Hennigan, 2020, n.p.). New York's Hart Island is the urban sprawl's "potter's field," a cemetery set aside normally to bury the unclaimed dead, indigents with no resources, and others who simply could not afford a funeral or cremation. Before the pandemic, Hart Island's staff of workers from the Department of Corrections in one week typically buried about 25 New Yorkers who fit the criteria; during the worst weeks of the pandemic, the team was burying 25 per day.

No one saw options. Funeral homes had no space in their refrigerators or even in the myriad of refrigerated trucks brought in to help with the overflow. Morgues in hospitals and the Medical Examiner's Office were filled beyond capacity, and people continued to die at astronomical rates. Frustrating and sad as it was, there simply seemed to be no alternative (Alsharif & Sanchez, 2021). One Pennsylvania funeral home owner 170 miles away tried to help his colleagues in New York City by cremating several bodies each week but although deeply appreciated, made only a small dent in the backlog. For New York's funeral profession, there was simply no way to keep up.

New York may have been the epicenter of the pandemic in the United States, but it was far from the only major community impacted. Italy's death toll in the early weeks of the pandemic exceeded that of every other country in the world. As a result, emergency health laws forbade funerals; undertakers like Massimo Mancastroppa were forced to do the best they could to serve families. Families of hospitalized patients had been unable to visit for days or weeks before death, and now the law restricted families from even seeing the body after death. Because in the early weeks of the pandemic, Italian officials believed clothing could harbor the virus, coffins were sealed immediately so the dead were buried in hospital gowns rather than their favorite suit or dress. Funeral directors were forbidden from placing letters or other memorabilia inside the casket as part of the sweeping restrictions, and when the cemeteries became too backlogged, the army stepped in to transport the dead to a crematory (Bettiza, 2020).

Although the Roman Catholic Church officially permits cremation, being forced by the state to have one's family member cremated without a funeral mass was the final indignity for many of the traditional faithful, especially in Italy's rural communities. In many cases, burials were held without even a blessing from a priest and were attended only by the undertaker. The most these funeral professionals were often able to do was send a photo of the casket to the family (Bettiza, 2020).

How Communities Responded in Funerals

More than three years after the pandemic began, one funeral celebrant sadly recalled the emptiness of funeral chapels equipped to seat 200 with only 8 or 10 family members in attendance for a service. When governments from nations to local jurisdictions around the world began enacting rules in the spring of 2020, the patchwork of regulations made it difficult to know what was acceptable behavior. The cemetery and funeral home where this celebrant regularly works was located in a jurisdiction that limited funerals fully and quickly, forbidding more than ten people to be gathered in one place even when the service was held outside, even when mourners maintained the obligatory six feet of physical distance between one another.

In a neighboring municipal cemetery, operating authorities enacted an even more stringent rule allowing a funeral director, a clergy member or other officiant, and a single family member to attend burials, a rule similar to the one depicted in the opening narrative of this chapter. The celebrant told of a particularly sad funeral on a rainy day. Because the cemetery had erected no tent or other shelter over the grave, rain poured off the top of the casket while the celebrant and the one family member did their best to honor the life of the deceased. Innumerable scholarly papers and news articles have chronicled the depth of funeral disruption wrought by the pandemic (MacNeil et al., 2023).

Even though deep distress at the restrictions on funerals for their loved ones was experienced by many families around the world (Boholano & Bacus, 2022; Júnior et al., 2020; Mas'amah et al., 2023), families and communities created myriad substitute grief rituals when they could not participate in the culturally bound rituals they had come to know. If the adage is true that "necessity is the mother of invention," the COVID-19 pandemic provided ample opportunity for families and communities to become "inventive" in the face of great "necessity."

Funeral homes that found a measure of success with one activity shared their best practices with others through networks and professional associations. One such creative idea was the popularization of "Hugs from Home," a system whereby individuals prohibited from or who simply preferred not to attend a funeral service in person could email a message to the funeral home whose staff, in turn, transcribed the message onto a card for the family. In several such applications of the idea, funeral directors then tied each card to a weighted helium-filled balloon to occupy one "seat" in an otherwise empty funeral chapel, greeting the handful of family members permitted to attend the ceremony.

Virtual funeral involvement played an extraordinarily important role in coping with the early chaos of grief for many families and communities. MacNeil and colleagues (2023) conducted a scoping review, initially considering more than 1,300 reports of the use of web-based media and social media in peer-reviewed journal articles, commentaries, and news reports. In many studies published thus far, families indicate some level of satisfaction with the ceremonies they created and, in some cases, even relish in the opportunities to have included more people than would have been able to travel to participate in a ceremony even before the pandemic.

One research respondent recalled the virtual funerals (plural) he created when his wife died suddenly in July 2020. Complicating the experience was that the widower and his wife had recently moved to the senior community where they resided when she died and many of their closest friends and extended family lived several hours away. "What we missed the most," he explained, "was the visitation where family members and friends get to share and hear stories."

The couple's minister recommended the funeral to be conducted in their church because it was such an important part of both of their lives, and the minister arranged an organist, a singer, and a single handbell ringer who would toll the bell at the appropriate times in the liturgy. Six or seven friends had prerecorded video tributes in which they told their favorite stories and these were used in an online gathering forum after the main funeral service had been concluded. A dozen or so family members, appropriately distanced from one another, sat in the pews in the front rows of the church and the entire service was webcast through the Zoom online teleconference platform. Only after the funeral was over did the grieving husband realize there were more than 350 computers logged on to the Zoom room, and with two or more individuals watching at many of those screens, he was overwhelmed at the response. "Those people were logged on from all over North America—the world, actually—and many of them could never have attended the funeral if we had conducted just a conventional service in the church at two o'clock in the afternoon," he noted.

Bitusikova (2020) reported a similar experience in reflecting on the death of a friend's mother. The traditional Jewish funeral service and shiva were required to be held entirely online because the jurisdiction where the mother died, coupled with her death from COVID-19 in the early days of the pandemic (when bodies were thought to be especially contagious), meant that neither family nor rabbi was allowed to be present for the burial. As the deceased's adult son explained, "It is about how you manage what's left . . . what agency you have" (p. 53).

In response to the restrictions, the family's rabbi led the gathered mourners in the traditional prayers that make up the burial rite, making sure that the funeral prayer book was available to participants. The texts remained visible to participants throughout the service. A few hours later, Bitusikova reported, many of the same individuals gathered for the virtual shiva. Even though the physical rituals of shiva were not shared between participants, many of the participants ate ceremonial foods in their own homes, covered mirrors, and lit candles. About the experience, Bitusikova concluded,

> The online participation in the funeral was about three-times higher than the closest family expected. Friends and relatives from all over the world who would otherwise be unable to attend due to various

reasons (illness, distance, finances, and so on) took part in the ceremony and had a place "in the first row."

(p. 53)

Although this chapter was written during the summer after the World Health Organization declared COVID-19 to no longer be a health emergency, it is still early and much data are more anecdotal than empirical. Nevertheless, reports of high levels of satisfaction about virtual funerals seem to have come mostly from individuals making up the "dominant" culture in high-income countries. Individuals who hold tightly to traditional cultural values, speak a language other than the dominant language of the community where they live, have limited access to or are irregular users of internet media, and who are part of low-resource families and communities have generally expressed far less satisfaction with the outcomes of virtual funeral ceremonies.

In their comparison qualitative study of pandemic funerals in Denmark and Australia, Gotved and colleagues (2023) found that funeral service had become far more "mediatized" during the pandemic, from the ways that funeral professionals communicate with each other and the public to the actual conduct of rituals. In the minds of the study authors, this "mediatization" of the funeral service profession simply follows a general social movement toward greater use of and reliance on media. Before the pandemic, Danish funeral professionals relied heavily on person-to-person interaction in planning rituals and carrying out the details of funerals. Media use was generally limited to a funeral home website, phones, and less frequently, a social media presence on sites such as Facebook.

Similarly, the study authors found that before the pandemic, Australian funeral directors relied on these technologies but heavily depended on personal interaction with families. The use of video screens for life tribute videos were commonly found in funeral homes before the pandemic, but only a few funeral providers possessed significant ability to livestream services. Although there were significant restrictions on gatherings, including physical distancing and restrictions on the number of people in attendance, in both Denmark's and Australia's government restrictions, funerals were seen as "essential events." Nevertheless, the significant restrictions on both indoor and outdoor events in Australia produced increased demand for livestreaming of services (pp. 111–112).

Funeral directors in other countries improvised in the same ways that their Australian and Danish colleagues did. Understandably, the use of technology expanded during the pandemic with much greater reliance on teleconferencing technology to meet with families and organize the details related to funeral ceremonies in the same ways that business meetings and school classes began to be conducted online through Zoom, Microsoft Teams, and similar platforms.

After restrictions were imposed on public gatherings in the spring of 2020, funeral homes that did not already possess equipment for streaming either resorted to someone in the family, a friend in attendance, or a funeral service staff member who held their mobile phone aloft and "streamed" the funeral, usually through Facebook Messenger or similar platforms. As the pandemic wore on, many American funeral homes invested in more permanent equipment with higher quality sound and video than could be captured on an individual mobile device.

Virtually all funeral professionals interviewed believe the streaming of funerals is a permanent change. Some believed that the ready availability of webcast services would reduce funeral attendance because it is so much more convenient to log on and watch rather than getting dressed up, taking off work, and driving to a location to be in person. At least anecdotally, these concerns appear unfounded since communities that were quickest to reduce restrictions have seen funeral attendance rebound to levels similar to those before the pandemic.

When mourners are mobility challenged or unable to travel long distances on short notice to attend a funeral, livestreamed services provide these mourners with an opportunity to view the service in real time, even if they cannot be physically present. What these mediated ceremonies do not provide, however, is the proximity of nearness, the ability to touch and be touched and to share a physical space with other mourners. This was particularly evident in the reports of interviewees in Gotved et al. (2023) who found that funeral director job satisfaction suffered most among those who treasured caring, in-person conversations with bereaved families but were unable to carry them on. One Danish funeral director noted that the "practical aspects of communication" could be handled via media. "But the absolutely, and equally important contact and communication in physical meetings, [the] hand shaking and showing of care and respect from one human to another, did change for the worse" (p. 113).

The assumption of funeral service professionals in interviews about the staying power of livestreamed funerals mirrors the research about religious service attendance in the United States. Although in-person worship attendance dropped significantly during the shutdowns of 2020 and 2021, many congregations anecdotally report larger in-person attendances in 2024 than in 2019. In tracking the same group of individuals' responses in a longitudinal survey of worship attendance from 2019 to 2022, 87% reported no change in their rates of worship attendance over that period. Of the remaining group who reported a change in their worship attendance habits, 4% reported they attended services more often and 8% reported they attended less. The researchers noted,

> The share of U.S. adults who take part in religious services in some way (in person, virtually or both) in a given month has remained

remarkably steady since the early days of the pandemic—even though *how* they participate has shifted dramatically.

(Nortey & Rotolo, 2023, para. 3)

Although the majority of congregations that began livestreaming their services during the early part of the pandemic have continued to do so, Nortey and Rotolo (2023) noted that in July 2020, 27% watched online or on TV, while in November 2022, only 12% of attendees reported watching services virtually.

White Evangelical Protestants have consistently led the religious communities with in-person worship attendance during the pandemic, but Black Protestants have experienced "a substantial bounce in physical attendance from a low of 14% in July 2020 to 41% (in November 2022)" (Nortey & Rotolo, 2023, para. 9). Worship community attendance is not a precise proxy for funeral attendance, but funeral service and clergy respondents indicate they often seem to move in similar directions.

Mental Health Consequences from the Pandemic

Grieving during the pandemic has proven to be fraught with complexities for bereaved families and communities. Social support is an essential element of healthy grieving, and the lack of social support during the pandemic led to what many clinicians and researchers noted early as increased levels of depression, anxiety, insomnia, stress, fear, and loneliness, and for some groups, suicide attempts increased during the early months of the pandemic. In the United States and some other countries, the rate of death by drug overdose climbed at a faster rate during the pandemic than in the years before (Appa et al., 2021; Hossain et al., 2020; Hoy & Harris, 2020; Júnior et al., 2020; Yard et al., 2021).

Opioid overdose deaths had been increasing annually when the pandemic struck, though circumstances surrounding the pandemic seems to have exacerbated the problem. Appa and colleagues (2021) conducted a cross-sectional analysis of opioid overdose deaths in San Francisco, California, comparing the 8.5 months before the shelter-in-place order was issued on March 17, 2020, finding that overdose deaths increased by 50% in the period after the stay-at-home order was issued. In their study, they found that the average age of the decedents did not change appreciably in the two study periods. They noted that although the proportion of Black decedents decreased slightly after the stay-at-home order, the overdose fatality rate remained significantly higher for the Black population (272 per 100,000 compared to 89 per 100,000 for whites). In April, May, June, July, and August, the number of opioid overdose deaths were from 150% to 300% higher than for the same months in 2019. Ironically, the researchers reported, 537 individuals died from opioid overdose between March 17 and November 30, an increase of 172 deaths over the pre-stay-at-home-order period. During the 8.5 months after the stay-at-home order was issued, 169 individuals died from COVID-19 (Appa et al., 2021, pp. 3–4).

In a cross-sectional study of nearly 190 million emergency department visits, Holland and colleagues (2021) found that visit rates for mental health conditions, suicide attempts, drug and opioid overdoses, intimate partner violence, and child abuse and neglect were higher in mid-March through October 2020, during the COVID-19 pandemic, compared with the same period in 2019. These findings were consistent with observations from other researchers (e.g., Yard, et al., 2021) who noted an increase in emergency department visits for child maltreatment and neglect.

Júnior and colleagues (2020) cited several studies and scholarly perspectives about the role and multiple benefits of funeral rituals for the mental well-being of the family. In their Brazilian context, they suggested that the inability of mourners during the pandemic to enact cultural funeral rituals "reinforces the painful nature of death . . . [and] amplifies and causes emotional trauma" (p. 3).

Yard and colleagues (2021) found that although emergency department visits for suicide attempts declined overall in the early months of the pandemic, there were significant increases of suspected suicides among some groups. For adolescent girls (aged 12–17), emergency department visits for suspected suicide attempts increased 26.2% during the summer of 2020 and were 50.6% higher during the winter of 2021 when compared to 2019's corresponding periods (p. 889). The study authors hypothesized these findings indicate severe distress among young females, though they cautioned that an increase in suicide attempts did not lead to an increased suicide rate during the early months of the pandemic.

In their study of rural Indonesian bereaved families during the pandemic, Mas'amah and colleagues (2023) found that the lack of appropriate funeral rituals—either because of restrictions or logistics—exacerbated the emotional pain experienced by family members after a loved one's death. However, their findings discovered another significant issue that dominates community beliefs. In the consensus belief of this community, the dead do affect the living, and when the dead do not receive appropriate ceremonies, their spirits wreak havoc on family members and the community. Neighbors were understandably frightened by the unritualized dead, leading to reports of blaming and shunning behavior from neighbors toward these newly bereaved families, presumably because these families somehow allowed their loved one to fall ill with the virus and because they did not provide adequate rituals in an effort to appease the dead.

Experiences in Italy echoed those from other studies around the globe. As noted earlier, Italy suffered some of the highest COVID-related mortality rates with few families and no community escaping its devastation. After their interviews with 40 respondents, researchers noted,

> Many families saw their loved ones get into an ambulance and never return, only to receive their ashes some time later. For most, no funerals could be organized and the bereaved were forbidden to find comfort in a friendly embrace because of the lockdown restrictions.
> (Testoni et al., 2021, p. 2)

While calling for patient analyses of the data and care in drawing quick conclusions about the effects of the pandemic, Burrell and Selman (2022) noted that funeral restrictions would likely contribute to increased mental health symptoms: "Qualitative research highlights the importance of meaningful and supportive funerals for the bereaved," and this is especially true among marginalized groups (p. 357). They called for continuing research to assess the impact of alternative ways individuals grieve and the modalities used for creating ceremonies in the face of death. "Becoming bereaved during COVID-19 presents challenges at every stage of the funeral process, from planning to post-funeral rituals and memorialization" (p. 358), noting that time and research that is both sensitive and methodologically robust will be required to fully assess the health effects on individuals and communities.

None of this is particularly surprising for those who have worked with bereaved people, assisted individuals through mental health issues, or helped bereaved families create personally meaningful funeral rituals (Hoy & Harris, 2020). In her work on complicated mourning, Rando (1993) noted the inestimable value of funeral rituals in the bereavement process: "For example, appropriately designed funerals are one of the best and potentially most therapeutic rituals available" (p. 313).

Clinical Implications

One of the essential elements funeral ceremonies provide is the surrounding of bereaved individuals with social support. Even for community members who are themselves grieving, the gathering together with others who are also mourning a death seems to provide a sense of solidarity in the loss and a mutual sense of support. Clinicians and other caregivers must be alert to any events—whether natural or human induced—that serve to prevent this all-important gathering in the face of grief. It follows from the research about social isolation and its likely impact on mental well-being that the lack of an opportunity for appropriate funeral rituals may lead to such mental health disturbances as complicated grief and even eventually prolonged grief disorder.

Clinicians and other caregivers can serve bereaved individuals well by inquiring about the funeral ceremonies that were available when their loved one died. If it is discovered that there was compromise in the hoped-for rituals and ceremonies, caregivers can inquire about details from bereaved individuals about what was missed and what the individual would have hoped to occur in the way of ceremonies.

As important, caregivers may wish to offer to help bereaved individuals create memorial rituals in the context of bereavement-focused counseling that serve as surrogate ceremonies. Incorporating the bereaved individual's ideal music, scripture, poetry, or other meaningful texts can make the ritual truly therapeutic. The sharing of photos and other memorabilia between the bereaved individual and the clinician can also prove helpful, especially when the bereaved person explains the significance of the items. A thoughtful and heartfelt eulogy can be an important addition to the ritual as well in which the bereaved individual writes out favorite stories and memories or recasts the deceased person's character and impact on the world.

This cocreated ritual can be conducted at the grave or other place of memorial meaning with the bereaved person's choice of family or friends. Alternatively, the ritual can be conducted in the therapist's office utilizing psychodrama (Worden, 2018, pp. 166–167), the Gestalt "empty chair" technique (Worden, 2018, p. 173), or simply as a ritual with the clinician quietly bearing witness to the pain of the loss. Even in his call for more personalized rituals for grief, Martin (2023) affirms the value of cultural customs: "Rather than jettison tradition altogether, there remains enormous value in tapping the collective wisdom of customs practiced around the world to inform the design of a personal grief ritual" (p. 85).

Reflection and Discussion

- What do you most remember about the suffering you and those around you endured during the COVID-19 pandemic?
- In what ways did reading the author's description of the pandemic's history rekindle traumatic memories for you?
- What was the most creative funeral expression you saw or read about during the pandemic?
- The author wrote from the perspective of four years after the pandemic began. How do you see the issues described here playing out in your community and among the people to whom you provide care?

References

Alsharif, M., & Sanchez, R. (2021, May 7). Bodies of COVID-19 victims are still stored in refrigerated trucks in NYC. *CNN*. https://www.cnn.com/2021/05/07/us/new-york-coronavirus-victims-refrigerated-trucks.

Appa, A., Rodda, L.N., Cawley, C., Zevin, B., Coffin, P.O., Gandhi, M., & Imbert, E. (2021). Drug overdose deaths before and after shelter-in-place orders during the COVID-19 pandemic in San Francisco. *JAMA Network Open*, 4(5), e2110452–e2110452. https://doi.org/10.1001/jamanetworkopen.2021.10452.

Bettiza, S. (2020, March 25). Coronavirus: How COVID-19 is denying dignity to the dead in Italy. *BBC World News*. https://www.bbc.com/news/health-52031539.

Bitusikova, A. (2020). COVID-19 and the funeral-by-Zoom. *Urbanities*, 10(4), 51–55.

Boholano, H.B., & Bacus, R.C. (2022). Catholic funeral traditions and alterations due to the COVID-19 pandemic: Implications to compliance to health protocols. *Journal of Positive School Psychology*, 6(6), 10614–10630. https://journalppw.com/index.php/jpsp/article/view/9688.

Burrell, A., & Selman, L.E. (2022). How do funeral practices impact bereaved relatives' mental health, grief and bereavement? A mixed methods review with implications for COVID-19. *Omega*, 85(2), 345–383. https://doi.org/10.1177/0030222820941296.

Feyman, Y., Avila, C.J., Auty, S., Mulugeta, M., Strombotne, K., Legler, A., & Griffith, K. (2023). Racial and ethnic disparities in excess mortality among U.S. veterans during the COVID-19 pandemic. *Health Services Research*, 58(3), 642–653. https://doi.org/10.1111/1475-6773.14112.

Gotved, S., Gould, H., & Klastrup, L. (2023). COVID-19 and the mediatization of the funeral industry in Australia and Denmark. *MedieKultur*, 38(73), 100–121. https://doi.org/10.7146/mk.v38i73.128439.

Hennigan, W.J. (2020, November 18). Lost in the pandemic: Inside New York City's mass graveyard on Hart Island. *Time*. https://time.com/5913151/hart-island-covid/.

Holland, K.M., Jones, C., Vivolo-Kantor, A.M., Idaikkadar, N., Zwald, M., Hoots, B., Yard, E., D'Inverno, A., Swedo, E., Chen, M.S., Petrosky, E., Board, A., Martinez, P., Stone, D. M., Law, R., Coletta, M.A., Adjemian, J., Thomas, C., Puddy, R.W., Peacock, G., . . . Houry, D. (2021). Trends in US emergency department visits for mental health, overdose, and violence outcomes before and during the COVID-19 pandemic. *JAMA Psychiatry*, 78(4), 372–379. https://doi.org/10.1001/jamapsychiatry.2020.4402.

Hossain, M.M., Tasnim, S., Sultana, A., Faizah, F., Mazumder, H., Zou, L., McKyer, E.L.J., Ahmed, H.U., & Ma, P. (2023). Epidimiology of mental health problems in COVID-19: A review. *F1000 Research*, 9(636), 1–16. https://doi.org/10.12688/41000research.24457.1.

Hoy, W.G., & Harris, H.W. (2020). Unintended consequences of COVID-19. *GriefPerspectives*, 19(3), 1–5. https://www.baylor.edu/medical_humanities/index.php?id=967441.

Jarden, R.J., Scott, S., Rickard, N., Long, K., Burke, S., Morrison, M., Mills, L., Barker, E., Sharma, K., & Twomey, B. (2023). Factors contributing to nurse resignation during COVID-19: A qualitative descriptive study. *Journal of Advanced Nursing*, 79(7), 2484–2501. https://doi.org/10.1111/jan.15596.

Júnior, G.J., Moreira, M.M., & Rolim Neto, M.L. (2020). Silent cries intensify the pain of the life that is ending: The COVID-19 is robbing families of the chance to say a final goodbye. *Frontiers in Psychiatry*, 11, 570773. https://doi.org/10.3389/fpsyt.2020.570773.

Kobo, O., Abramov, D., Fudim, M., Sharma, G., Bang, V., Deshpande, A., Wadhera, R.K., & Mamas, M.A. (2023). Has the first year of the COVID-19 pandemic reversed the trends in CV mortality between 1999 and 2019 in the United States? *European Heart Journal: Quality of Care and Clinical Outcomes*, 9(4), 367–376. https://doi.org/10.1093/ehjqcco/qcac080.

MacNeil, A., Findlay, B., Bimman, R., Hocking, T., Barclay, T., & Ho, J. (2023). Exploring the use of virtual funerals during the COVID-19 pandemic: A scoping review. *Omega: Journal of Death and Dying*, 88(2), 425–448. https://doi.org/10.1177/00302228211045288.

Martin, P.M. (2023). *Personal grief rituals: Creating unique expressions of loss and meaningful acts of mourning in clinical or private settings*. Routledge.

Martyr, P. (2023). Australian Catholics' lived experiences of COVID-19 church closures. *Journal of Religion and Health*, 62, 2881–2898. https://doi.org/10.1007/s10943-023-01826-6.

Mas'amah, A.A.A., Bunga, B.N., Liem, A., & Kiling, I.Y. (2023). Death, funeral rituals, and stigma: Perspectives from mortuary workers and bereaved families. *Pastoral Psychology*, 72(2), 305–316. https://doi.org/10.1007/s11089-022-01053-9.

Nafilyan, V., Islam, N., Mathur, R., Ayoubkhani, D., Banerjee, A., Glickman, M., Humberstone, B., Diamond, I., & Khunti, K. (2021). Ethnic differences in COVID-19 mortality during the first two waves of the coronavirus pandemic: A nationwide cohort study of 29 million adults in England. *European Journal of Epidemiology*, 36(6), 605–617. https://doi.org/10.1007/s10654-021-00765-1.

Nortey, J., & Rotolo, M. (2023, March 28). *How the pandemic has affected attendance at U.S. religious services*. Pew Research Center. https://www.pewresearch.org.

Pathirathna, M.L., Nandasena, H.M.R.K.G., Atapattu, A.M.M.P., & Weeraskara, I. (2022). Impact of the COVID-19 pandemic on suicidal attempts and death rates: A systematic review. *BMC Psychiatry, 22*(506), 1–15. https://doi.org/10.1186/s12888-022-04158-w.

Rando, T.A. (1993). *Treatment of complicated mourning*. Research Press.

Reyes, C., Husain, N. Gutowski, C., St. Clair, S., & Pratt, G.R. (2020, April 7). Chicago's coronavirus disparity: Black Chicagoans are dying at nearly six times the rate of white residents, data show. *Chicago Tribune*. https://www.chicagotribune.com.

Selman, L.E., Chao, D., Sowden, R., Marshall, S., Chamberlain, C., & Koffman, J. (2020). Bereavement support on the frontline of COVID-19: Recommendations for hospital clinicians. *Journal of Pain and Symptom Management*, 60(2), e81–e86. https://doi.org/10.1016/j.jpainsymman.2020.04.024.

Testoni, I., Azzola, C., Tribbia, N., Biancalani, G., Iacona, E., Orkibi, H., & Azoulay, B. (2021). The COVID-19 disappeared: From traumatic to ambiguous loss and the role of the internet for the bereaved in Italy. *Frontiers in Psychiatry*, 12, 620583–620583. https://doi.org/10.3389/fpsyt.2021.620583.

U.S. Center for Disease Control and Prevention. (2023). CDC museum COVID-19 timeline. https://www.cdc.gov/museum/timeline/covid19.html.

U.S. Department of Health and Human Services. (2023). Bulletin: Civil Rights, HIPAA, and the Coronavirus Disease 2019 (COVID-19). https://www.hhs.gov/sites/default/files/ocr-bulletin-3-28-20.pdf.

Worden, J.W. (2018). *Grief counseling and grief therapy: A handbook for the mental health practitioner* (5th ed.). Springer.

World Health Organization. (2023, May 5). Statement on the fifteenth meeting of the IHR (2005) emergency committee on the COVID-19 pandemic. https://www.who.int/news.

Xia, Z., & Stewart, K. (2023). A counterfactual analysis of opioid-involved deaths during the COVID-19 pandemic using a spatiotemporal random forest modeling approach. *Health & Place*, 80, 102986–102986. https://doi.org/10.1016/j.healthplace.2023.102986.

Yard, E., Radhakrishnan, L., Ballesteros, M.F., Sheppard, M., Gates, A., Stein, Z., Hartnett, K., Kite-Powell, A., Rodgers, L., Adjemian, J., Ehlman, D.C., Holland, K., Idaikkadar, N., Ivey-Stephenson, A., Martinez, P., Law, R., & Stone, D.M. (2021). Emergency department visits for suspected suicide attempts among person aged 12–25 years before and during the COVID-19 pandemic—United States, January 2019–May 2021. *Morbidity and Mortality Weekly Report*, 70 (24), 888–894.

Chapter 8

Honoring the Homegoing

African American Experiences with Funerals

Undoubtedly, many people "attended" their first African American funeral by viewing the rites for Grammy-winning recording artist Whitney Houston on February 18, 2012. More than 8 million people watched the funeral ceremony either through the live television broadcast or internet connection, telecast from the New Jersey church where Houston grew up and where her singing career got its start. Thousands of onlookers stood on nearby streets surrounding New Hope Baptist Church as an all-star cast of entertainers, politicians, recording executives, family members, and close friends eulogized the 48-year-old singer. Cable News Network (CNN) reported that a peak 5.4 million viewers visited its website to view the live telecast of the event, a number approximately ten times its usual Saturday afternoon viewership (Stelter, 2012). Several video reproductions of the entire 3-hour, 34-minute funeral reside on the internet; one reproduction on the video-sharing site YouTube had more than 2.2 million views in the first nine months after the singer's death (Wesawthat1, 2012).

Celebrity funerals attract large numbers of people to both broadcasts and to the live events themselves, even if these people cannot get into the venue where the service is held. Crowds numbering in the millions lined processional routes and viewed media accounts of funeral rites for President John F. Kennedy, Princess Diana, and entertainer Michael Jackson, clearly demonstrating that people whose lives have been touched by a celebrity sense a need to gather with concerned others in the face of that individual's death (Hoy, 2013). When the decision was announced that Houston's funeral would be an invitation-only affair rather than a Michael Jackson–like memorial service at a venue such as Newark's Prudential Center, the choice was seen by many fans as a "slight" (Star-Ledger Staff, 2012).

Eight years later, a global audience was once again riveted to televisions and computer screens to watch an African American funeral. Only this time, the ceremony was for a man previously unknown outside his family and friendship network. A few days before this service, George Floyd had been restrained and killed at the hands of four Minneapolis police officers, a crime for which the officers involved were eventually

DOI: 10.4324/9781003353010-9

tried, convicted, and sentenced to prison (Levenson & Kirkos, 2022). Like the Grammy-winning Houston's service, Floyd's was watched by millions, with the four-hour service carried by every major broadcast network and widely available online.

For people without such renown, African American funerals, commonly referred to as "homegoings," share many characteristics in common with these two frequently viewed ceremonies. Together, these ceremonies provide important reference points for those who might be unfamiliar with these customs (Na & Hoy, 2015). To explain customs to those who care for African American families, this chapter provides what ethnographers call "thick description" (Geertz, 1973) of customs from enumerable settings and studies that both describe observations and catalog the meanings assigned to these ceremonies by a diversity of African American mourners, clergy, and funeral service professionals.

From Celebrity to Unknown: Commonly Observed Practices

Because of her celebrity status, Houston's death and funeral garnered wide media attention, drawing reporters from news and entertainment organizations around the world. African American funeral director respondents indicate the rites were "typical" of Black funerals in the United States except for the "all-star cast" (Hoy, 2013, 2016, 2021, 2022; Na & Hoy, 2015). In a similar vein, George Floyd's homegoing ceremony also garnered wide media attention and an all-star cast. However, these participants were generally drawn from individuals who spoke to the circumstances of Floyd's death rather than his celebrity status. Usually, African American funerals are characterized by speakers representing friends and family, traditional religious or other music favored by the deceased, scripture readings, prayers, and a eulogy delivered by the deceased's pastor or other minister. Although funerals do not typically include words and music delivered by Hollywood celebrities like Dionne Warwick, Tyler Perry, and Kevin Costner (as in the case of Whitney Houston's funeral), nor by political leaders and civil rights activists such as now-president Joe Biden and the Reverend Al Sharpton (as in the case of George Floyd's funeral), they do usually feature speakers and musicians who are well known to the deceased and the bereaved family.

Death and Homegoing in African American Experiences

The notion of homegoing is a time-honored construct among African American communities that contrasts the spiritual (generally Christian) views of a happy, immortal life in heaven with the emotional realities of a mortal existence characterized by suffering and oppression. In the African American tradition, ministers often begin funerals with words such as

"Welcome to this homegoing celebration" and then go on to explain the Christian meaning of the term (Graham, 2002). Printed materials at these funerals are often characterized by the title "Homegoing" on the cover with a color photo of the deceased, usually in vigor and good health. In recent years, one might have observed the addition of airbrushed angel wings and halos that are superimposed onto the studio portrait of the deceased person, adding to the spiritual notion of homegoing.

In reviewing the history of African American funeral directing, Smith (2010) noted that the criticism leveled at funerals in general in the United States in the mid-20th century by authors such as Mitford (1963) failed to consider the deep traditions shared among African Americans to honor loved ones in death when they had been denied such honor in life. Smith's analysis is joined by others such as Raboteau (2004) who have demonstrated the importance of triumphalism in slave homegoing ceremonies that has carried over to contemporary culture. African American customs developing in the early part of the century included such rituals as "settin' up" with the deceased at a wake with an open casket, spirited music, multiple eulogies, and a sumptuous meal where stories and memories were shared (Smith, 2010, pp. 83–87).

Funeral traditions among African Americans are historically rich and culturally significant, and these customs are not recent in their development. A former slave himself and at the time president of Tuskegee Institute, Booker T. Washington (1907) wrote about the unique African American view:

> The great mystery of death has given the ceremonies that are connected with this dread event a special and peculiarly important place in their social life. Out of this instinctive awe and reverence for the dead has arisen the demand for solemn and decent and often elaborate burial services.
>
> (p. 94)

A common feature among these services is the holding in tension the bereaved family's deep experience with loss with jubilant thanksgiving for a "way of escape," a resolved assurance that the deceased has now "gone home" and away from the difficulties of the present world. In his retrospective of his career in cross-cultural bereavement research, Rosenblatt (2017) noted that "in the 1970s, I was strongly inclined to think that all humans grieve in rather the same way. Now I am sure I was wrong" (p. 618).

Rosenblatt's retrospective is important in that his work was among the earliest applications of ethnography to bereavement. One significant contribution to the literature on African American grieving is the notion that bereavement is socially constructed, meaning that ideas and definitions of such terms as "grief," "mourning," "feeling," and "religion" are shaped by their own sociocultural environment (Rosenblatt, 2001).

Funerals have long been regarded as a potentially significant element in a family's and community's ability to cope with grief following the death of a loved one. In the fifth edition of the landmark textbook on grief counseling, Worden (2018) offered the same evaluation in precisely the same words he had written in the first edition more than 35 years earlier and in every intervening edition as well:

> The funeral service has come in for considerable criticism, especially after the 1984 report of the Federal Trade Commission. But the funeral service, if it is done well, can be an important adjunct in aiding and abetting the healthy resolution of grief.
>
> (p. 120)

Most often connected to the deceased's religious background, the notion of homegoing in African American communities honors the difficulties with which individuals have struggled throughout history. In spite of the constitutional abolishment of slavery in 1865, African Americans have continued to face high burdens of disease, mistreatment, and early death. The notion of homegoing has reminded family and community that the best life is that which occurs *after* death as individuals are reunited with their Creator and their deceased relatives and friends to live in a blissful paradise, a perfect "home" (Barrett & Heller, 2002; Holloway, 2003; Smith, 2010).

The notion of escape from the travails of life in a world of injustice is ancient. The Christian faith frequently recites the words of its first-century spokesman, Paul of Tarsus, when he wrote, "For to me to live is Christ, and to die is gain" (Philippians 1:21, KJV). Nineteen centuries later, the words were echoed by African American statesman, W.E.B. DuBois (1903/2003), when, following the death of his son, he acknowledged the mixed emotions with which he viewed the death. He experienced his own nearly embarrassing "gladness of heart" as he reflected on the freedom of his son not having to live in a world of deep discrimination: "My soul whispers ever to me, saying 'Not dead, not dead, but escaped; not bond, but free'" (p. 151).

In one of the earliest attempts to differentiate death and bereavement issues between cultural groups, Kalish and Reynolds (1981) articulated differences between their urban Black American, Japanese American, Mexican American, and Anglo-American respondents. Most African Americans in Kalish and Reynolds's study of 200 respondents reported they looked to friends and church members in addition to reliance on family members.

Rosenblatt and Wallace (2005) interviewed 26 bereaved African American individuals, finding that the respondents held a belief of high emotionality of African American grief when compared to European American grief. Moreover, approximately half of the respondents indicated they believed racism played an important role in their loved one's death, leading to feelings of anger, rage, and frustration about racial injustice in addition to the frequently reported bereavement emotions of sadness or loneliness.

Bordere's (2008) phenomenological study of ten young African American adolescent males in New Orleans provides perspective on how young people see funerals. In interviews, these young men described the general helpfulness they garnered from participating in both the "regular funerals" (usually in a church or funeral home chapel) and the "second line" jazz portion of the funeral that is characteristic of New Orleans. Participating in the music, movement, and dance that are common in such second-line experiences provided a means for these young men to express their sense of loss, literally acting out their experience with loss.

Burns (2011) has written an exhaustive history of the funeral of Dr. Martin Luther King Jr., a paradigm for African American funerals in the 1960s. King's funeral was transformed from purely psychosocial-spiritual consolatory ritual into an opportunity for civic discourse. Burns described both the content of the funeral itself and the context for the ceremony, pointing out the features that honored King's personal investment and contribution in the cause of civil rights and the choice to have his simple casket borne on a mule-drawn farm wagon. The idea of the funeral as an opportunity for civic discourse is explored more fully in Chapter 2 of this volume.

Anchoring the Mourning Process in the Funeral Experience

The five anchors described in Chapter 1 are evident in African American homegoing celebrations, such as Whitney Houston's, George Floyd's, and the other lesser-known decedents whose services have been studied. Significant symbols, gathered community, ritual action, connection to cultural heritage, and transition of the body are all vital in these ceremonies. While each anchor is interpreted against the backdrop of the spiritual homegoing ideal, the format provides an organizing framework to help outsiders better understand African American mourning.

Significant Symbols

Like those of many other groups, African American funerals are generally replete with significant symbols, including flowers, photos, life celebration videos, and the ubiquitous religious symbols appropriate to the deceased's or family's faith community. Some of these symbols will be obvious to any observer while others, such as the selection of Whitney Houston's favored lavender roses in floral arrangements, are much more subtle and perhaps known only to intimates.

Custom portrait art is common at African American funerals. At the front of the church for George Floyd's homegoing service stood two easels with identical large artistic portraits of him, each with airbrushed angelic wings and halo. In her funeral home selection room near a wide variety of caskets, one African American funeral director displayed sample items from which a family could choose to incorporate the deceased's photograph. Using a photo provided by the family, an artist would design a customized blanket, wall tapestry, or head panel for the inside of the casket. The funeral director explained that these items provided an important memorial keepsake for those families who chose to utilize them.

Gathered Community

African American community members generally turn out en masse for a funeral, demonstrating the anchor of gathered community. Na and Hoy's (2015) grounded theory study of video recordings of African American homegoing ceremonies found that 100% of the recordings provided evidence of virtually full churches and funeral home chapels with almost no empty seats. One of the most devastating aspects of the COVID-19 pandemic on African American funeral customs was the restriction on these gathered events (Palmer, 2022), a concern considered more thoroughly in Chapter 7.

The gathering of community in the face of death is vital to the Black funeral experience according to interviewed funeral directors and published research about African American funeral experiences. Unlike the custom frequently seen among European Americans, who most often bury or cremate their dead within a few days, African American funerals will often be delayed by a week or more to allow time for extended family to gather from far and wide (Armstrong, 2010; Barrett, 1995; Collins & Doolittle, 2006; Hoy, 2022; Smith, 2010).

For African Americans, gathering has not always been either legal or safe. Throughout the decades of American slavery, extending into the Jim Crow era of the early 20th century and culminating in the civil rights struggles of the 1960s, many whites saw the assembly of Blacks as synonymous with insurrection, protest, and revolt. In the antebellum South, slaveholders often allowed funerals for slaves to only be held at night when work did not have to be stopped, but even then, slaveholders were often highly suspicious of the "plans" being made by slaves under the auspices of commemorating their dead (Smith, 2010).

Gathering in the face of grief is a custom as old as time itself. The attempts by some European Americans in the mid-20th century to reduce or entirely eliminate gatherings in their own cultural customs in an attempt to "simplify" the funeral is a practice not in evidence in African American communities. Rather, African Americans join with the vast majority of the world's groups in gathering for funeral rituals, declaring to bereaved family members and the larger community, "We will not let you walk this road alone."

Ritual Action

Ritual actions are the specific activities undertaken by mourners to help them "join in the action" of the funeral. As explained in Chapter 1, this is literally where mourners "walk out what they cannot talk out." Whether placing candles and balloons at the entrance to Newark's New Hope Baptist Church, signing any of dozens of "memorial register books" set up around the world, or writing a letter to place on the impromptu memorial outside the Beverly Hilton Hotel, grieving fans responded to Whitney Houston's death in the same ways bereaved people have responded since the beginning of recorded history—through active participation in rituals to express the emotional and spiritual impact of the loss.

African American funeral customs have involved mourners in a diversity of tasks throughout their history. Historian Suzanne E. Smith (2010) declared,

> The African American slave funeral from the colonial era through the antebellum period was one of the most central ways the slave community was able to assert its essential humanity. In colonial times, the funeral ceremony allowed many recently enslaved Africans to honor their heritage and practice religious rituals that gave them a sense of connection to their homeland.
>
> (p. 25)

She went on to write, "The slave funeral served as the foundation of several key elements of African American life, including the early origins of an independent Black church, the organization of mutual aid and burial societies, and ultimately—through the establishment of the funeral industry—a very successful form of Black entrepreneurship" (p. 26).

In the West African homeland of North American slaves, members of the family and community moved into action immediately after the death of a loved one; the funeral provided ample opportunity for the involvement of many in the tasks of burying the dead (Armstrong, 2010; Barrett, 1995; Smith, 2010). Celebrity funerals provide a unique challenge to mourners' desires to be involved, however, because so many tasks are professionalized, with the sheer number of grieving people far outnumbering the tasks to be accomplished.

Connection to Cultural Heritage

The anchor of connection to cultural heritage was summarized well by Barrett (1995), who wrote,

> The unique and colorful character of the Black church is a byproduct of the African American interpretation of the Western church and, as with traditional West African funeral rites, the normative practice of African American funeral rites is significantly related to religious beliefs.
>
> (p. 81)

Many of the distinctives of African American homegoing ceremonies illustrate the role of culture and are explained more fully below. Scripture that is both read and recited provides a primary focus during African American homegoing ceremonies. Moreover, spirited music, cadence in movement, "call and response" during the eulogy, and the prolific use of professional cars are all illustrative of the role of culture in these ceremonies.

Transition of the Body

Integral in the North American Black funeral tradition is the role of the corpse, illustrating the anchor of transition of the body. Whereas some North Americans of Western European descent have sought to remove the body from the funeral service and create what Long (2009) called "disembodied funerals," African American families and communities have largely resisted those changes (Collins & Doolittle, 2006; Glass & Samuel, 2011; O'Meara, 2004; Smith, 2010).

"Appropriate" disposition of the body is a high value throughout African American communities (Barrett, 1995; Collins & Doolittle, 2006; Smith, 2002; Smith, 2010; Stow, 2010). In interviews during and after the COVID-19 pandemic, African American funeral directors indicated that relatively few families chose cremation and virtually all prefer funeral rites with the body present when they were permitted to make those choices. When restrictions were relaxed, mourners returned to their pre-pandemic funeral choices. Although cremation and funerals without the body present are more widely accepted among younger African Americans than older segments of the population, cremation is still not accepted nearly as widely as with European Americans (Buchanan & Gabriel, 2015; Glass & Samuel, 2011; O'Meara, 2004).

Even though the funeral homes visited in person and online display an array of caskets in a broad range of prices, funeral directors and bereaved individuals report that the least expensive models are rarely chosen and that families often opt for pricey customizations, such as having a name engraved on the lid of a casket or having a photo collage airbrushed into a customized head panel. African Americans seem to place a high level of emphasis on the role of the deceased body in funeral ceremonies. Na and Hoy (2015) found every funeral they studied included the presence of a casketed body, a finding corroborated by Buchanan and Gabriel (2015, p. 31) in their study of 510 university students, which found that 23.1% of African American students surveyed would consider cremation in contrast to 60.5% of white students.

Features of African American Homegoing Experiences

Although all five of the ceremonial anchors are evidently important in African American homegoing experiences, the distinctives become clear in the anchors of cultural connection and body transition. In her compelling prologue to a history of African American funeral directing, Smith (2010) wrote that for African Americans, funerals have never been just about honoring the dead or somehow appeasing their spirits to prevent them from bothering the living. During the period of transatlantic slave trade as they gathered in "hush harbors" to acknowledge their dead, "African Americans first began to use funerals to both bury their dead and plan a path to freedom. In African American culture, death was never simply the end of life and funerals were never simply occasions to mourn" (p. 14).

Multiple researchers have noted that African American funerals employ a diversity of culturally appropriate and sometimes unique customs to help family members and community members create meaning in the face of death (Barrett, 1995; Holloway, 2003; Hoy, 2022; Na & Hoy, 2015; Rosenblatt & Wallace, 2005; Smith, 2010). Surveys, researcher observations, and qualitative interviews with bereaved family members and caregiving professionals have traditionally made up the bulk of data from which ethnographers draw what they call "thick descriptions" of cultural groups.

In recent years, cross-cultural funeral researchers have been helped by the ready availability of entire funerals via online video-sharing services such as YouTube and Vimeo. One widely acknowledged ethnographic problem arises when researchers are not insiders to a particular culture in that one's presence in the ceremony potentially changes the behavior of group participants. Although researchers who view funerals via video are limited by the camera angles available, an ethnographic research advantage is achieved by outsiders not changing the actions of the actors (Na & Hoy, 2015).

The following distinctive tools illustrate some of the ways African American families and communities create meaning in the face of death by arranging and participating in homegoing ceremonies.

Vital Role of the Faith Community

In one of the deepest studies recently completed on Black American religious experience, Mohamed and colleagues (2021) surveyed more than 8,600 African Americans across generations, supplemented by small-group discussions with survey respondents and interviews with African American clergy. Funerals are not the only time when faith communities play a central role in African American experiences:

> Religion has long figured prominently in the lives of Black Americans. When segregation was the law of the land, Black churches—and later, mosques—served as important spaces for racial solidarity and civic activity, and faith more broadly was a source of hope and inspiration.
>
> (p. 8)

They further found that more than 70% of African American adults born before 1965 attend church regularly (pp. 3, 14), so it is little surprise that the faith community's role would figure prominently into funeral customs.

Mohamed et al.'s (2021) findings may provide explanation to Holloway's (2003) conclusion that church traditions largely dictate the differences between white funerals and Black funerals. Among the common elements Na and Hoy (2015) found in their research of African American funeral ceremonies, four of the six had direct connection to the spiritual aspects of the service: the funeral's setting in the church or connected with church people, the extensive use of scripture, the centrality of preaching (eulogy), and the use of gospel music. These findings were echoed several years later in a broader study on economic aspects of funerals in African American communities (Hoy, 2022).

Levin et al. (2005) as well as Taylor et al. (2014) have reported a consistent and predictable sense of supportiveness among African Americans from their church; 81.2% reported attending church at least a few times each year. Interviews with African American funeral directors and clergy indicate that religious faith has generally been thought to be important for bereaved African American families even when they may not have been actively involved in a religious community before the loss.

In the studies of Sharpe and Boyas (2011) and Sharpe and Iwamoto (2022), these culturally bound sources of comfort and support may contribute to reductions of post-traumatic stress disorder (PTSD) among African American homicide survivors. In one study, for example, Sharpe and Boyas (2011) found that African American survivors of homicide utilized spiritual support and meaning making, maintained a connection with the deceased (often through some kind of linking object), coped and cared for others through a collective initiative, and tended to conceal emotions from others in order to cope with their grief. This iterative process tends to employ cultural and psychosocial resources for coping with some of the most horrific experiences. Although the study found that bereaved African American homicide survivors tended to rely more on personal spiritual coping strategies (e.g., personal prayer) than on communal spiritual resources (e.g., church attendance), these results must be interpreted cautiously when relating them to funerals since these respondents were months to years along in their loss experiences.

Primacy of Scripture

From the beginning of a Christian African American homegoing service until its end, the sacred words of the faith are paramount, apparently even for individuals who were not actively engaged in a faith community or who may not have been overt in their practice of the faith's traditions. Although Mohamed and colleagues (2021) found nearly 50% of young African Americans (born after 1981) seldom/never attend church, funeral directors and clergy respondents indicate that the vast majority, even among this group, looks to traditional customs of Christian faith when their parents and contemporaries die, with the notable exception being those individuals and families who practice Islam (Hoy, 2022).

Christian African American funerals usually begin with various quotations from the Bible including well-loved passages from Psalms, quoted from memory by clergy as they lead family into the church from the back door to the family's designated seats. Readings from the Old Testament and the New Testament are frequently highlighted in the opening minutes of the funeral ceremony, and the lead clergy's "eulogy" (funeral sermon) almost always employs innumerable allusions to and direct quotations from scripture.

The Reverend Dr. Rufus Wright recited five passages from the Old Testament book of Psalms from memory as he led the family into the Fountain of Praise Church for George Floyd's homegoing. The Christian scriptures were significantly involved in the remainder of the service as well. Biblical allusions embedded in music, sermonic reflections on scripture within the eulogy, and the near ubiquitous Old Testament and New Testament readings were present in this ceremony, as they are in other African American homegoing ceremonies observed in prior research. In the 27 African American funeral ceremonies observed by Na and Hoy (2015), all but one included the recital of scripture, including many of the passages recited by Dr. Wright in opening Floyd's service.

In addition to the spirited gospel music that was part of Whitney Houston's homegoing, the funeral was filled with prayers, scripture, and allusions to Houston's homegoing. The largest single segment of the service was a 25-minute-long rhythmic eulogy (sermon) delivered by Rev.

Marvin Winans, who frequently encouraged the gathered mourners to respond with "Amen" and "Hallelujah." Winans noted early in his remarks that attorneys had called him inquiring if he wanted to protect the intellectual property rights in his sermon. "I don't know how I can do that," he explained to the mourners, "because I'm going to preach the Word. This is not a speech; I'm going to preach." Affirming the heritage of Christian faith evident in Houston's family, Winans thanked the entertainer's mother for scheduling the funeral at New Hope Baptist, "bringing the world to church today" (Wesawthat1, 2012).

In one funeral observed by Na and Hoy (2015), the 22-minute eulogy delivered by the pastor included more than 40 direct quotes or references to scripture. Either in explaining the quoted scripture or offering theological premises, funeral speakers tend to reference God's care and protection in the midst of suffering. In several African American funerals for homicide victims, themes of God's concern for justice and the Christian imperative for love to overcome racism can also be observed.

Spirited Music Reflecting the Christian Message

Homegoing services are generally characterized by spirited music with many of the musical selections coming from the same traditional Christian gospel genre that might be heard on Sunday in an African American church. Observers of African American homegoings whose own traditions are different often remark about the amount of time given to music, the presence of musical interludes or "background" to speakers, and the highly spirited tone of music.

Music is frequently accented by syncopated rhythms, with crescendos building from quiet interludes to intense expressions of praise to God. Observers will notice both family members and other attendees singing along, clapping, and moving to the beat of the music following the lead of soloists, instrumental musicians, and ensemble members. This apparent "jubilation" seems paradoxical to the otherwise expected solemnity of a funeral service, especially when a young person has died.

Lyrics of the chosen songs are frequently punctuated with words like "hallelujah," "praise," and "amen," echoing the Christian message of hope heard in the scripture and eulogy with lines such as "You are the strength, of my life, You are the strength of my life, . . . it is well with my soul, hallelujah; You'll be lifted high, I surrender to your way, Oh God" (Smallwood, 2014).

George Floyd's homegoing service included a family viewing before family members were seated. In the last eight minutes of the family's final viewing before the casket was closed, the tone of the music clearly shifted from what had been quiet, reflective selections to a highly syncopated, rhythmic tune titled, "He'll Welcome Me" (Kee, 1995). Like much of the other music during the ceremony, the upbeat tune inspired family members and others to move to the beat of the music, clap their hands, and sing along with the musicians. The presentation of "Welcome Me" lasted for almost 8½ minutes, included a soloist, with the support of an ensemble, singing about the future day when the believer in Christ is "welcomed home" by Jesus and the others who have died before (C-SPAN, 2020, 39:00). The song opened with this verse:

> I'm living this life just to live again
> And with the Lord I know that I shall reign;
> I shall not stray, with Him I'll stay,
> Oh, He'll welcome His children home one day.
> (Kee, 1995)

"Resolutions" from Community Groups

Groups and individuals frequently participate in homegoing services by creating carefully crafted "resolutions" to be read aloud and given to the bereaved family. These resolutions are often written in elegantly scripted calligraphy on parchment paper and then read during the service by the "church clerk" or another woman in the congregation. The resolutions that were read and referred to at George Floyd's homegoing point to the large number of individuals engaged in the ritual action of crafting these acknowledgments (Hoy, 2013). Apparently, resolutions are written by one or more individuals who has been assigned the task by the community group sending the resolution. Sometimes resolutions are read during the funeral by representatives of the groups who sent them.

Although the exact history of the resolution custom is unknown, one African American funeral director from Ohio interviewed in conjunction with an earlier study said that resolutions were already a staple part of the African American funeral experience when he started practice in the mid-1950s. This funeral director speculated that the tradition "got legs" during a period of great poverty among African Americans when the "white custom" of sending flowers would have been far out of reach for many Black individuals, churches, and community groups.

These resolutions are typically written in legal-sounding language punctuated with "whereas" and "be it resolved." They will often lay out three or four paragraphs. The following is a fictitious example of such a resolution, created to illustrate the discoveries made in Na and Hoy's (2015) research:

> WHEREAS, our Eternal God has seen fit to call from this life His servant, Dorothy C. Smith, and WHEREAS we know the loss that surely must envelope her family, and WHEREAS, Sister Smith served the

> Lord faithfully as a wife, mother, grandmother, and friend, THEREFORE BE IT RESOLVED that the Pastor, Deacons, and members of the New Mt. Mariah Missionary Baptist Church do hereby declare our support for Sister Smith's family with our faithful prayers and offers of comfort from our Lord. BE IT FURTHER RESOLVED that a copy of this resolution shall be presented to the family and a copy kept in the permanent records of the New Mt. Mariah Missionary Baptist Church.
>
> (Na & Hoy, 2015, n.p.)

The service for George Floyd featured the complete reading of three resolutions; the officiants also acknowledged about 15 other resolutions by the name of their senders and referred to "countless others" that time did not permit them to name or read (C-SPAN, 2020, 1:21:32). Na and Hoy (2015) noted in their study many services when gathered mourners were told the number of resolutions sent was too numerous to read them all, and so a few had been selected to be read. At one such homegoing ceremony for a 32-year-old woman who had died from cancer, as each group's resolution was read, members of the sending group in attendance rose and stood silently as the resolution was read by a leader from the community group who sent the resolution.

Solemnity and Cadence

African American funerals are often characterized by somber cadences, high-stepping marches, and slow, deliberate movements, all adding a level solemnity to an already somber occasion. In the cases observed by Na and Hoy (2015), family members were led into the church or funeral chapel by a minister in a slow, deliberate procession as the homegoing service began.

The funeral for George Floyd included the high "stepping" of the senior funeral director as he led the procession of funeral service staff to the front of the church just ahead of the family's entrance (C-SPAN, 2020, 11:37), a symbolic gesture that is common albeit not universal. Interestingly, funeral director research participants were evenly split on the appropriateness of this custom with some sensing it was an important part of the highly choreographed African American funeral experience, while another group thought the custom to be, in the words of one respondent, "needlessly showy" (Hoy, 2022).

In many African American funerals, the casket is ceremonially closed soon after the beginning of the service once the family has had an opportunity to view the deceased and has been formally seated by the funeral service staff. When the casket is closed, it is most often done with great solemnity and deliberation. In one funeral, for example, the "closing of the bier" (as it was announced in the order of service printed in the memorial brochure provided to attendees) was a deliberate ceremony that lasted almost six minutes and included four funeral home staff members solemnly approaching the casket, two abreast, down the center aisle from the back of the church. The casket itself was closed slowly.

In some communities, it has become popular for eight trained pallbearers to hoist the casket to their shoulders at the end of the service, creating a final act of departure as they carry the casket past the mourners and ahead of the family to exit the church to the waiting hearse. In some cases, this is a memorial option disclosed on the funeral home's General Price List, with names such as "elite burial guard." In the 2020 funeral for George Floyd, this final act of departure added a solemn coda to what had been an elegant homegoing (C-SPAN, 2020, 4:20:14). Whitney Houston's funeral featured the hoisting of her casket onto the shoulders of a ceremonial group from the nearby New York Police Department.

Bordere's (2008) observations of the "second line" funerals in New Orleans are another example of how cadence and dance are woven into the funeral ritual for some African Americans. Traditionally, New Orleans jazz funerals have been characterized by slow, deliberate music and cadences on the way to the grave site, followed by jubilant dancing and upbeat music after the burial and the mourners are "cut loose".

Participatory Environment

The homegoing for George Floyd was a deeply participatory service. In addition to family members who spoke, 17 invited speakers, 11 musical soloists, and a cast of other musicians participated in the service. Additionally, the "call and response" of African American worship can be heard throughout the ceremonies as people called out "Amen," "Hallelujah," and "Preach it," common responses by congregants during the preaching in traditional African American Evangelical Protestant and Pentecostal worship services (LaRue, 2000). The homegoings for George Floyd, Whitney Houston, and others demonstrated many opportunities for participants to sing as a congregation, to offer verbal affirmation of the speakers, and to stand and rhythmically move with music.

Although not observed at the conclusion of either Whitney Houston's or George Floyd's homegoing, a common element observed by Na and Hoy (2015) and Hoy (2022) is the presence of flower bearers who carry flower arrangements out of the church behind the casket and family at the conclusion of the homegoing. The bearers tend to be women and girls from the congregation who seem specifically chosen to bear the flowers out to the waiting flower car. According to clergy informants, being chosen for this duty carries the same honor as having been chosen as a pallbearer to carry the casket.

Role of Professional Automobiles

Limousines for family members and other service participants also figure prominently into the symbolic role of funerals among African Americans (Barrett, 1995; Collins & Doolittle, 2006). Funeral directors say that most white-owned American funeral homes have reduced the number of limousines or eliminated them altogether from their fleets, but Black-owned funeral homes maintain several cars to be used when requested. The use of multiple limousines at a single funeral, while increasing the cost to bereaved families, is viewed as symbols of status and expressions to the world that the deceased was "somebody special," according to one African American funeral home owner.

Research demonstrates that photos of professional automobile fleets are frequently featured on the websites of African American–owned funeral homes and rarely on the websites of white-owned funeral establishments. In a random selection of funeral home websites, Hoy (2022) found that professional cars were featured prominently on the websites of 80% of African American firms and none of the European American–owned firms. In a visit to one funeral home, the owner invited me to step with her into the garage where she proudly showed her gleaming burgundy fleet of hearses, limousines, vans, and other professional vehicles estimated to be valued at more than US$2 million.

Centrality of the Casketed Deceased

Glass and Samuel (2011) reported significant discrepancies between the endorsement of cremation among their white and Black research participants. Among older Blacks, for example, 7% endorsed acceptance of cremation for oneself, while 73% of whites endorsed the choice. The discrepancy was not as pronounced among middle-aged adults, but among that group, 50% of middle-aged whites found the process acceptable while 27% of middle-aged Blacks found the process acceptable for oneself. The researchers noted, "Strongly-stated opinions against cremation were even more prevalent, particularly among the African American middle-aged adults" (p. 377). This observation is important because this is the group most likely to select funeral options for their older parents.

In their case study of one African American family from Kentucky, Collins and Doolittle (2006) wrote,

> A ceremonial and cultural aspect of African American funerals is to bury loved ones in a style benefitting a person of high esteem and importance. The funeral costs and final funeral arrangements embody a level of elegance that communicate that "somebody important has died."
> (p. 965)

Despite the fact that African American households have the lowest median income and highest rate of poverty of any ethnic group in the United States, Collins and Doolittle (2006) went on to explain, "The amount of money spent on the casket, limousines, and other funeral services make a statement about families' departed loved ones and signify the families' desire to give the deceased a 'fine and proper burial'" (p. 965).

Customs calling for a "fine funeral" run deep in African American history. Armstrong (2010) noted that African funerals demonstrated the cohesiveness of families and communities, citing the historical work of Franklin and Moss (2000). "Inasmuch as Africans believe that how they treat their dead will affect their quality of life, final rites are of utmost importance. Consequently, extensive and expensive death rituals are commonly accepted as the 'sacred obligations of survivors'" (p. 87).

Across North America, rites without the body present such as a direct cremation could certainly be arranged more economically than those that demand embalming, caskets, hearses, and limousines. Although this notion is amplified in Chapter 5, what makes "rational economic sense" to some outsiders seems, for many African Americans, to devalue the role of ceremony in the life of the family and community.

According to one research respondent who owns a direct-to-consumer crematorium, a "direct cremation" (with no viewing or services) could be arranged in his establishment for approximately 20% of the amount required for a "typical" traditional funeral in his community, but almost none of his clientele come from the nearly 25% of his county's population who are African American (Hoy, 2022). Clearly, some value is at play in these circumstances other than the simple economic maxim of "buy what is cheapest." To suggest that people should forgo customs with ancient roots and significant contemporary meaning in the interest of economics is clearly a Caucasian-centric perspective.

As is the case with most celebrities, the funeral for Whitney Houston likely did not create financial hardship for her family or estate. Several funeral directors interviewed identified the casket used for Houston as similar to the custom-made bronze models used for entertainers Michael Jackson and James Brown, purported at the time to cost between US $25,000 and US$30,000 (Russell, 2009). During the funeral service at New Hope Baptist Church, Houston's casket lay prominently positioned in front of the church's massive pulpit at the end of a wide center aisle.

In the video footage of the funeral service, musicians and speakers frequently gestured toward and looked directly at the casket as they spoke, a process that would have been undoubtedly more difficult without the presence of the casketed body and its unmistakable reminder of life and death. Kevin Costner changed "voice" in his eulogy from third person, where he talked *about* Whitney Houston, to second person, where he talked directly *to* the entertainer, a phenomenon previously analyzed by Kunkel and Dennis (2003). Near the end of his eulogy, Costner looked down from the pulpit to Houston's casket lying in front of the church and continued, "So off you go, Whitney, off you go, escorted by an army of angels to your Heavenly Father. And when you sing before Him, don't you worry—you'll be good enough" (Wesawthat1, 2012, 1:18:39).

The body of George Floyd was casketed in a heavyweight polished bronze casket with 14-karat gold-plated hardware, a model that Batesville Casket Company calls the Promethean (Z94). Batesville representatives and funeral directors confirmed it is the same casket model used for the funerals of Michael Jackson, Aretha Franklin, and James Brown. At the time of George Floyd's funeral, an online search showed the casket available in funeral homes at prices ranging from US$24,000 to $38,000.

Floyd's body was prominently displayed during the funeral; the casket was open for the family viewing as each person or group in the family made their way to the casket, presumably to say a final goodbye. When the camera angle permitted it, one could see several mourners making the Catholic sign of the cross or other gesture of respect as they stood in front of the open casket. This final viewing by family members lasted for nearly 28 minutes and was prominently featured at the beginning of the funeral.

After the viewing by the family was completed, funeral home staff tucked in the navy-blue velvet lining of the casket and closed the casket in a very deliberate, reverent, and dignified manner. From the moment funeral directors started lowering the lid until it came to rest on the casket rim was 26 seconds. For the remainder of the service, the closed casket rested as the focal center of attention in the front center of the church, a few feet from the immediate family (C-SPAN, 2020, 44:40).

Following the eulogy, eight members of the funeral home's elite burial guard made a cadenced and deliberate procession down the center aisle into the church. The funeral staff appeared to be unhurried even though the homegoing ceremony had already lasted for more than four hours. Upon reaching the front of the church, the elite burial guard members took their places around the casket and then, in a single motion, hoisted George Floyd's casketed body onto their shoulders, turned with his feet toward the door, and deliberately made their way from the church, swaying in cadence to the strains of Zac Cortez singing, "I Shall Wear a Crown" (C-SPAN, 2020, 4:20:14). In the camera angle from the back of the church, dozens of mourners could be seen holding up their smartphones to capture the procession on video.

"The More Things Change, the More They Stay the Same": The Future of Funerals in African American Communities

Scholars of cultural customs generally avoid engaging in prediction about the choices that will be made by future generations of specific social groups. Nevertheless, history is a good guide to understanding how societies make collective decisions, and virtually all mortuary anthropologists and funeral historians agree that funeral customs tend to change at a glacially slow pace (Hoy et al., 2021; Laderman, 2003; Metcalf & Huntington, 1991; Smith, 2010).

Without doubt, the landscape of funerals continues to change across North America and around the world. Interestingly, however, African Americans who could find "simpler" and "more economical ways" to memorialize their dead have proven resistant to European American, economically driven changes. Cultural customs bear influence and meaning that are not easily quantified in rational economic analysis (Hoy, 2013); see Chapter 5 of this volume for a deeper explanation of this phenomenon.

The homegoing ceremonies for George Floyd and Whitney Houston, as well as the ceremonies held for African Americans of less renown presage much of what is happening in the funeral landscape. First, funerals have already become very personalized, a trend likely to continue. Perhaps the influence of the baby boom generation and an increasing desire to find meaning in ritual lead bereaved families and communities to continue making adaptations to their death rituals. Some of this customization will be obvious, such as playing a recording of Whitney Houston's blockbuster hit "I Will Always Love You" as pallbearers carried her casket from the church.

Through the speakers who are chosen to represent the family and the deceased, through highly customized printed memorial programs replete with color photos, or through simpler photograph collages and "life tribute videos" shown to mourners at funeral gatherings, bereaved survivors will undoubtedly continue to embrace an effort to tell the deceased's life story through the funeral ceremony. When faith had been integral to the life of the deceased, undoubtedly spiritual symbols and words will abound in the funeral, especially notable in the themes of eulogies, chosen scriptures, and music selections. On the other hand, when faith was not central to the deceased's life, there will likely be less willingness on the part of family members to pretend otherwise by organizing a big church funeral, replacing it instead with a ceremony more in keeping with the deceased's values.

Second, like many ethnic communities, African Americans, as a group, will likely be very slow to jettison the traditional church funeral. One African American funeral director said that among his Black clientele, church funerals are still the leading preference. "Everybody wants a Christian funeral," he said, even if such choices require enlisting the help of a church the deceased never attended and the leadership of a minister the deceased never met (Hoy, 2016).

Despite cultural tastes and preferences, economic realities will likely persist for years to come. African American funeral directors noted the general refusal of families to endorse "simple cremation" but also pointed out that contemporary families more frequently choose only one limousine instead of the two, three, or four that might have been expected a decade ago. Families are concerned about funeral costs, one funeral director explained, but they still want funerals "with all the trimmings. When we show them what is available for less money," he continued, "most often, they opt for their first [and more expensive] choice anyway." Although community members may come to the aid of a family by hosting car washes and bake sales or simply by making cash contributions, according to the African American funeral directors interviewed, few families complain about costs or seemingly struggle to pay the funeral bill.

Clinical Implications

Professionals and volunteers who care for bereaved African American individuals, families, and communities will want to be alert to the importance the funeral or homegoing will play or may have played in the experience of a loved one's death. Asking questions about customs utilized and their personal meaning can help bereavement counselors become culturally attuned learners (see Chapter 3), an especially important characteristic for caregivers who are not of the ethnicity of the bereaved individuals they seek to help.

Clinicians must also be alert to financial constraints while recognizing the importance for culturally appropriate ceremonies that may not look "economically practical" to the outsider. Even cultural insiders often struggle with this dichotomy. One clergy informant explained that he tries to help families "think responsibly and as Christian stewards" but acknowledged that his advice is rarely heeded by bereaved families, who instead choose elaborate ceremonies, sometimes beyond what he believes they can easily afford. Cultural sensitivity demands that caregiving professionals maintain extreme caution in making recommendations to families about "simpler alternatives."

From their perspective as social workers, Glass and Samuel (2011, p. 373) recommend that their colleagues become well educated about memorial options in order to provide information to older adults and their families. Although these authors suggest that cremation options should be discussed with families, especially when finances are of a concern (p. 385), all professionals must proceed carefully when suggesting to families that they consider abandoning family history, custom, and tradition in exchange for monetary savings. Several bereaved family and professional informants indicated that community members rally around needy families to help pay for the funeral (Hoy, 2022), a custom also seen in contemporary sub-Saharan African people groups like the Luo of western Kenya (Hoy, 2013).

Collins and Doolittle (2006 shared the social workers' perspective but suggested that African American families with limited economic resources often incur costly funerals as a way to reclaim dignity and honor denied to the deceased in a society hostile to their ethnic heritage. They urged extreme caution for colleagues:

> Rather than look upon these practices as excessive, inappropriate, or in poor taste, professional helpers can use their understanding and knowledge of these funeral customs to reach out to families during their greatest moment of need and to provide technical and supportive assistance that is worthwhile to clients.
>
> (p. 966)

An individualistic "have it your way" approach might make "rational sense" in a worldview that highly prizes individual autonomy. However, when divorced from a strong understanding of family and collectivist cultural norms, such advice greatly risks intensifying family conflict and feelings of personal shame among the very people professionals seek to assist.

Most important from a cultural standpoint, celebrity funerals clearly remind the world that when a person has touched the lives of others, even anonymous others unknown to the decedent or family, the death of that individual needs to be honored and remembered, perhaps in ways that transcend the "practical," economically justified choices that critics of funeral ceremonies propose. Most of all, African American homegoing ceremonies remind the world's citizens that people arrange funeral ceremonies to meet a diversity of emotional and spiritual needs and attempt to create meaning in the face of sometimes unspeakable tragedy. No amount of seeming rationality is effective in talking people out of following their hearts.

Reflection and Discussion

- If you are not African American or if these customs are foreign to your own deathways, what tradition would you consider employing in your own funeral? Why do you find this custom significant?
- What factors in American slavery and contemporary poverty for many African Americans do you think are most significant for the development and continuance of these traditions?
- How do you respond to the idea that families might emotionally overspend?

References

Armstrong, T.D. (2010). African and African American traditions in America. In L. Bregman (Ed.), *Religion, death, and dying—Volume 3: Bereavement and death rituals* (pp. 83–109). Praeger.

Barrett, R.K. (1995). Contemporary African American funeral rites and traditions. In L.A. Despelder & A.L. Strickland (Eds.), *The path ahead: Readings in death and dying* (pp. 80–92). Mayfield.

Barrett, R.K., & Heller, K.S. (2002). Death and dying in the Black experience. *Journal of Palliative Medicine*, 5(5), 793–799.

Bordere, T. (2008). "To look at death another way": Black teenage males' perspectives on second-lines and regular funerals in New Orleans. *Omega: Journal of Death and Dying*, 58(3), 213–232. https://doi.org/10.2190/OM.58.3.d.

Buchanan, T., & Gabriel, P. (2015). Race differences in acceptance of cremation: Religion, Durkheim, and death in the African American community. *Social Compass*, 62(1), 22–42. https://www.doi.org/10.1177/0037768614560949.

Burns, R. (2011). *Burial for a king: Martin Luther King's funeral and the week that transformed Atlanta and rocked the nation*. Scribner.

Collins, W.L., & Doolittle, A. (2006). Personal reflections of funeral rituals and spirituality in a Kentucky African American family. *Death Studies*, 30, 957–969.

C-SPAN. (2020, June 9). George Floyd funeral service in Houston. https://www.c-span.org/video/?472882-1/george-floyd-funeral-service-houston#.

DuBois, W.E.B. (2003). *The souls of Black folk*. Barnes & Noble. Originally published 1903.

Franklin, J.H., & Moss, A. (2000). *From slavery to freedom: A history of African Americans* (8th ed.). Knopf.

Geertz, C. (1973). *The interpretation of cultures: Selected essays*. Basic Books.

Glass, A.P., & Samuel, L.F. (2011). A comparison of attitudes about cremation among Black and white middle-aged and older adults. *Journal of Gerontological Social Work*, 54(4), 372–389.

Graham, R.L. (2002). *I have a testimony: A perspective of death, grief and widowhood in African American culture* (Publication 3049166) [Unpublished doctoral dissertation]. University of North Carolina–Greensboro. ProQuest Dissertations Publishing.

Holloway, K.F.C. (2003). *Passed on: African American mourning stories*. Duke University Press.

Hoy, W.G. (2013). *Do funerals matter? The purposes and practices of death rituals in global perspective*. Routledge.

Hoy, W.G. (2016, April 14). *"Goin' up yonder": Death and meaning in African American eulogies*. Paper presented at the Association for Death Education and Counseling, Minneapolis.

Hoy, W.G. (2021, April 15). *Understanding homegoing: African American funeral experiences*. [Video file.] Pacific Northwest University of Health Sciences (Yakima, WA). https://pnwu.hosted.panopto.com/Panopto/Pages/Viewer.aspx?id=c39e2eb8-73de-4e8c-aae4-ad0b0160af1f.

Hoy, W.G. (2022, April 22). *African American funeral choice: The role of cultural customs and economic means*. Paper presented at the Association for Death Education and Counseling, St. Louis, MO.

Hoy, W.G., Becker, C.B., & Holloway, M.L. (2021). Memorialization and death-related rituals. In H.L. Servaty-Seib & H.S. Chapple (Eds.), *Handbook of thanatology: The essential body of knowledge for the study of death, dying, and bereavement* (3rd ed.; pp. 207–234). Association for Death Education and Counseling.

Kalish, R.A., & Reynolds, D.K. (1981). *Death and ethnicity: A psychocultural study*. Baywood.

Kee, J.P. (1995). He'll welcome me. [Song]. *Show up!*Bridge Building Music.

Kunkel, A., & Dennis, M.R. (2003). Grief consolation in eulogy rhetoric: An integrative framework. *Death Studies*, 27, 1–38. http://dx.doi.org/10.1080/07481180302872.

Laderman, G. (2003). *Rest in peace: A cultural history of death and the funeral home in twentieth-century America*. Oxford University Press.

LaRue, C.J. (2000). *The heart of Black preaching*. John Knox Press.

Levenson, E., & Kirkos, B. (2022, July 27). Two ex-officers who restrained George Floyd sentenced to three years and 3.5 years in federal prison. *CNN*. https://www.cnn.com/2022/07/27/us/tou-thao-kueng-george-floyd-sentence/index.html.

Levin, J., Chatters, L.M., & Taylor, R.J. (2005). Religion, health and medicine in African Americans: Implications for physicians. *Journal of the National Medical Association*, 97(2), 237–249.

Long, T.G. (2009). *Accompany them with singing: The Christian funeral*. Westminster John Knox Press.

Metcalf, P., & Huntington, R. (1991). *Celebrations of death: The anthropology of mortuary ritual*. Cambridge University Press.

Mitford, J. (1963). *The American way of death*. Simon & Schuster.

Mohamed, B., Cox, K., Diamant, J., & Gecewicz, C. (2021, February 16). *Faith among Black Americans*. Pew Research Center. https://www.pewresearch.org/religion/2021/02/16/faith-among-black-americans/.

Na, Y., & Hoy, W.G. (2015, April). *Examining video to clarify African American funeral experiences*. Paper presented at the Association for Death Education and Counseling, San Antonio.

O'Meara, B. (2004). *Study of American attitudes toward ritualization and memorialization: 2005 update*. Wirthlin Worldwide. http://www.ogr.org/documents/WirthlinReport2005_001.pdf.

Palmer. B. (2022). American homegoing: On the richness of the Black funeral tradition. *Virginia Quarterly Review*, 98(3), 134–159.

Raboteau, A.J. (2004). *Slave religion: The "invisible institution" in the antebellum South*. Oxford University Press.

Rosenblatt, P.C. (2001). A social constructionist perspective on cultural differences in grief. In M.S. Stroebe, R.O. Hansson, W. Strobe, & H. Schut (Eds.), *Handbook of bereavement research: Consequences, coping, and care* (pp. 285–300). American Psychological Association.

Rosenblatt, P.C. (2017). Researching grief: Cultural, relational, and individual possibilities. *Journal of Loss & Trauma*, 22(8), 617–630. https://doi.org/10.1080/15325024.2017.1388347.

Rosenblatt, P.C., & Wallace, B.R. (2005). *African American grief*. Routledge.

Russell, J. (2009, July 9). Batesville Casket is coy about starring role in Jackson funeral. *USA Today*. http://usatoday30.usatoday.com/money/industries/manufacturing/2009-07-09-michael-jackson-casket_N.htm.

Sharpe, T.L., & Boyas, J. (2011). We fall down: The African American experience of coping with the homicide of a loved one. *Journal of Black Studies*, 42, 855–873. https://doi.org/10.1177/0021934710377613.

Sharpe, T.L., & Iwamoto, D.K. (2022). Psychosocial aspects of coping that predict post-traumatic stress disorder for African American survivors of homicide victims. *Preventive Medicine*, 165, 10277. https://doi.org/10.1016/j.ypmed.2022.107277.

Smallwood, R. (2014) Total praise. [Song.]*WOW 2000s*. Sparrow Records.

Smith, S.E. (2010). *To serve the living: Funeral directors and the African American way of death*. Belknap.

Smith, S.H. (2002). "Fret no more my child . . . for I'm all over heaven all day": Religious beliefs in the bereavement of African American, middle-aged daughters coping with the death of an elderly mother. *Death Studies*, 26, 309–323.

Star-Ledger Staff. (2012, February 17). Speculation over Whitney Houston private family viewing grows. *Star-Ledger*. http://www.nj.com/news/index.ssf/2012/02/speculation_over_whitey_housto.html.

Stelter, B. (2012, February 21). Whitney Houston funeral drew millions on TV and online. *New York Times*. http://www.nytimes.com/.

Stow, S. (2010). Agonistic homegoing: Frederick Douglass, Joseph Lowery, and the democratic value of African American public mourning. *American Political Science Review*, 104(4), 681–697.

Taylor, R.J., Chatters, L.M., & Brown, R.K. (2014). African American religious participation. *Review of Religious Research*, 56(4), 513–538. https://doi.org/10.1007/s13644-013-0144-z.

Washington, B.T. (1907). *The Negro in business*. Hertel, Jenkins. https://openlibrary.org/works/OL357524W/The_Negro_in_business.

Wesawthat1. (2012). *Whitney Elisabeth Houston funeral service 18 February 2012 Newark, New Jersey*. [Video.] http://www.youtube.com/watch?v=yqq-V134aO8.

Worden, J.W. (2018). *Grief counseling and grief therapy: A handbook for the mental health practitioner* (5th ed.). Springer.

Chapter 9

Memorial Ceremonies

Where We Have Been, Where We Are Going

The trip to Kisumu was uneventful in every way as we exchanged funds from U.S. dollars to Kenyan shillings, purchased medicine and supplies, and began our return trip to the Nyakach Plateau. Here each summer, groups of professors and students from Baylor University worked with nonprofit Straw to Bread and its grassroots Kenyan counterpart, Bethlehem Home. As we traveled in our group's *matatu*, a 12-passenger minivan, southeast along County Road A1 toward Ahero, we came upon a unique sight for the Americans traveling in our group.

Driving at about 60 kilometers per hour was another *matatu* with no fewer than 20 passengers, who sang and clapped as they traveled. But atop this minibus was a gold-colored human casket, tied to the top of the van with several ropes. It appeared that the bereaved family inside the *matatu* was accompanying their recently deceased relative home to the family compound where the funeral would commence that Friday afternoon. If that family followed other Luo customs I have observed (Hoy, 2013), they would host 100–300 friends and extended family members for an all-night observance of mourning, dancing, singing, and feasting. Then the funeral experience would culminate the following day with a Christian ceremony and a burial of the casketed body in a grave dug by men in the community.

The centerpiece of the entire event would be the dead body in an open casket. If this family's experience was like others I have observed, the casket would be set up under its own canopy near where the family and friends would gather in their all-night vigil and feast. Knowing that many Luo families struggle to host this culturally expected ritual, I inquired of our working-class truck driver about his family's customs. After he confirmed for me that the last time there was a death in his family, the funeral customs were similar to what I had observed, I asked him casually, "I see there is a crematorium in Kisumu. Would your family consider cremating the body to save money?" With what I perceived to be a look of incredulity on his face, his reply was direct: "Of course not. We respect our dead."

DOI: 10.4324/9781003353010-10

The costs of a funeral is a favored explanation for why customs for memorialization have changed in some groups and among some families. Undoubtedly, there is truth to that assertion for some families, as discussed in Chapter 5. However, the changes that are occurring in family choices in funeral ceremonies seem to be less driven by costs and more driven by other factors. Some bereaved individuals, for example, expect to move from their current community and so they seem less connected to the community cemetery where perhaps several generations of ancestors are buried.

Concern about the "waste" of cemetery space and wanting to be a proper steward of the land has led some others to choose natural burial options without embalming chemicals, metal caskets, and cemetery vaults. A few have begun embracing options such as human composting, where the body is passed through a system that leads to rapid decomposition and the family receives a cubic yard of mulch at the end of the process.

At the beginning of the 21st century, the majority of those not choosing earth burial chose cremation, a process during which the body is heated to a high temperature and then the pulverized bone fragments are returned to the family. For religious communities such as Hindus and some Buddhists, the practice of cremation is seen as a freeing of the spirit from the body. Many bereaved individuals who do not observe the beliefs and practices of these faith communities also see great spiritual meaning in cremation.

Cremation is almost always the final disposition for those who make the philanthropic decision to have the entire body donated to medical science and research after death. In those cases, once the body has served its teaching or research purposes, the remains are cremated, and those cremated remains are returned to the family. More recently, some have developed other means of disposing of the dead body including alkaline hydrolysis or water cremation. Whether the disposition becomes part of the memorial ceremonies, bereaved families and communities often ascribe significant meaning in the choices about what becomes of the corpse.

What Do We Do with the Corpse?

The fifth of the anchors of memorial ceremonies presented in Chapter 1 is "transition of the corpse." Although the mode of disposing of the body does not always impact the kind of ceremony chosen, there can be significant connections. In their study of death rituals reported by parents after intensive care unit pediatric deaths, Brooten and colleagues (2016) noted that choices about what to do with the remains and in what kind of rituals to engage were deeply related to the parents' cultural background and to the parents' financial resources. One parent reported cremating the child's body because "I just couldn't bear to put my son in the ground and have the worms eat him up," while another said, "I'm Catholic, so I don't believe in cremation. . . . If I want to burn, I will burn in hell" (p. 136). The researchers concluded that parental decisions related to memorial ceremonies were both stressful and complex.

Burial of the body in the earth has long been regarded as the "traditional" mode of disposition of the corpse in the West. Because the Abrahamic religions of Judaism, Christianity, and Islam have historically preferred earth burial, cultural groups whose beliefs are influenced by these religious systems have tended to practice customs that open a space in the soil, deposit the body there, and then cover the corpse with the earth that was removed to make the hole.

For some, the deceased body is wrapped in linen or wool fabric and placed in the ground. Among the Luo of western Kenya, older interview informants recalled a time when their grandparents were buried wrapped in one or more leaves from the banana tree. British colonization made coffins widely available by the mid-20th century, and virtually all Luo are now buried in Western-style caskets made of wood or metal. The story that opened this chapter is just such an example of how ancient cultural customs are often adapted to incorporate new symbols, like a casket for the body.

Although the earliest known use of burial coffins to enclose the body date back at least 10,000 years to the Neolithic period in China (Australian Museum, 2018), the most notable Chinese burial is that of Lady Dai, a noblewoman who died in Hunan Province in 163 B.C.E. In her ornate multichambered tomb accidentally discovered when workers were excavating a bomb shelter in 1971, the 2,100-year-old mummified remains were accompanied by more than 1,000 artifacts apparently placed in the tomb to accompany the deceased into a pleasant afterlife. Her perfectly preserved body was found inside the innermost of four nested lacquered coffins, dressed in a silk gown embroidered with dogwood flowers. Each hand held a silk sachet filled with spices, flowers, and fragrant reeds (Bonn-Muller, 2009).

Although many other East Asian people groups almost exclusively cremate their dead, early 21st -century Chinese bereaved families chose earth burial in equal proportion until 2018, when a slight majority of Chinese families began choosing cremation (CEIC Data, 2023). The Taoist custom of Qingming (tomb-sweeping day) is an important festival for many Chinese families as they demonstrate filial piety through the burning of bamboo paper made to resemble money as well as paper cars and jewelry in order to provide goods to their ancestors (Liu, 2022).

Historically, a coffin to enclose the dead body was seen as a demonstration of wealth, and only the aristocracy could afford one. Saqqara is an ancient Egyptian burial site dating from about 650 B.C.E. and located south of Cairo. Speaking about the 100 elaborately decorated wooden coffins recently found there, archaeologist Ramadan Hussein noted that the cemetery served a wealthy city of priests and government officials: "The richness of the city at the time is reflected in the richness of the burials" (Curry, 2020, n.p.).

In the United States, like in much of the West, declining preference for earth burial and a consequent rise in the cremation rate mean that fewer families overall choose earth burial. Nevertheless, funeral directors who serve large numbers of African Americans, Latin American immigrants, and African immigrants confirm that earth burial is highly preferred among these populations. These preferences echo the choices made by immigrants in their countries of origin. In Mexico, for example, the proportion of decedents whose remains were cremated rather than buried rose during the COVID-19 pandemic, though earth burial remains the overwhelming choice. In 2019, 8.7% of decedents were cremated, and in 2020, the percentage rose to 11.8% (CE Noticias Financieras, 2020). Some evidence demonstrates that cremation was common in prehistoric Mexico but that the practice was prohibited by the Spanish conquerors, likely due to their Roman Catholic beliefs and customs (Ramos-de Viesca et al., 2002).

Cremation has been practiced in India for more than two millennia among Buddhists, Hindus, Jains, and eventually Sikhs (Prothero, 2001). Although Western assumptions are that Indian Hindus always cremate their dead, Arnold (2016) cited public health data from 1880, when only 43% of Hindus in Bombay were cremated, as an example. Among the lower castes of India, burial was usually chosen, most likely because of the high cost of wood for a ceremonial cremation; however, as the 19th century progressed, "Hindus, regardless of caste, chose to follow the prestigious rite of open-air cremation" (p. 401). Famines and epidemics seemed to have raised the proportion of decedents who were cremated, and in most cases, those changes have become permanent.

In the West and in most urban centers outside of India, open-air cremation pyres have been replaced by crematoriums that employ natural gas or, less often, electric retorts to cremate bodies. A modern crematory's retort will quickly reach temperatures of 1,400–1,600 °F (760– 870 °C), allowing a body's fat and water content to burn off to gases, leaving only bone fragments behind. In contemporary Western crematoriums, following the cremation, the bone fragments are then pulverized into smaller, generally unrecognizable fragments called cremated remains (Cremation Association of North America, 2023a).

Contemporary Western proponents of cremation often argued that the process was an "environmentally friendly" way to dispose of the dead because when not used for cemeteries, the land could be used more effectively. However, as Arnold (2016) pointed out, "in India cremation was a fuel-hungry, polluting technology that bore considerable environmental costs" (p. 398). One of the arguments against cremation in the 21st century is that even with efficient natural gas cremators, the carbon footprint of cremation is significant, contributing its own share to climate change (Hager, 2023, Kelly, 2015).

Some ancient Europeans also practiced cremation. Even though some kind of rudimentary embalming (likely using honey) was common and bodies of deceased warriors were "laid out" for viewing, ancient Greeks likely also introduced cremation to the West in 1000 B.C.E. Homer's epics indicate that soldiers were frequently buried quickly on the battlefield, but at least in some cases, warriors were cremated near the place of their death when they died far from home to enable their remains to be transported back to families in the homeland (Mylonas, 1948).

Although cremation has been practiced among Hindus for centuries, the first crematorium in Europe opened in 1876 in Milan, after a law was enacted two years earlier that made cremation legal in Italy. Almost simultaneously, an American crematory opened in Washington, D.C., but its facilities were much less ritual-oriented than its European counterpart. Crematoriums almost always included a space for ritual service (mourning halls); therefore, they became places where services were conducted and concluded with the cremation of the body in the presence of the family and other mourners. As some found these "witnessed cremations" to be highly objectionable, the ritual sites and the technical aspects of cremation were separated, sometimes even into separate buildings. Meanwhile, designers and owners seemingly made great efforts to camouflage chimneys and furnaces, hiding them from public view (Dlábiková et al., 2022).

When the first German crematorium opened in Gotha in 1878, bodies were placed on a catafalque for the ceremony in the funerary hall. At the conclusion of the ceremony, bodies were sent along a rail system to the basement and into the gas-fired cremation chamber. Somewhat over an hour later when the cremation was finished, the cremated remains were returned in an urn to the family waiting in the funerary hall (Dlábiková et al., 2022, p. 28).

In their tracing of the history of cremation, Dlábiková and colleagues (2022) noted that the acceptance of cremation was highly varied among different people groups. Cremation became acceptable in many majority-Catholic communities only after the Roman Catholic Church changed its doctrine to accept cremation in 1963, citing the need to preserve land for the living.

The Cremation Society of England was established in 1874, five years before the first crematory opened. The society's membership agreement declared its members' belief in cremation:

> We disapprove the present custom of burying the dead, and desire to substitute some mode which shall rapidly resolve the body into its component elements by a process which cannot offend the living and shall render the remains absolutely innocuous.
>
> (Thompson, 1891, p. 7)

Cremation, like burial and the other "disposition options," is not a substitute for ceremonies. If a family chooses cremation but wants a traditional funeral with viewing, many funeral directors will accommodate the request by use of a ceremonial or rental casket. Such products include a reusable outer "shell" of wood or polished metal and a removable insert in which the deceased body lies for the visitation, viewing, and funeral service; afterward, the removable insert is cremated with the deceased. Rutherford (2001) found this to be an especially attractive option for Catholic families for whom the Church prefers the entire body be brought to church for the funeral liturgy (mass). Such options also potentially save a bereaved family money since the family is essentially renting a casket.

Whether a bereaved family chooses to hold a "traditional funeral" with the body present followed by cremation or chooses to hold a memorial gathering without the body, cremation may provide more options for families in their memorial choices. Without a decaying corpse to be disposed of, cremation affords families the option of delaying public ceremonies until "a more convenient time," perhaps weeks or months after the death. Typically, a burial accompanies the funeral ceremony, frequently as the ceremony's last component. Cremation, on the other hand, affords more flexibility with scheduling because the cremated remains can be retained indefinitely to be present at the memorial service in the future.

A preference for simple ceremonies does not necessarily imply a choice for cremation since some individuals object to cremation for emotional and environmental reasons. For some, the thought of burning the remains of their loved ones is far more objectionable than placing the body in the ground. The Catholic dad quoted earlier in this chapter is an example of the emotional and spiritual toll cremation can take on a bereaved individual or family when they find such treatment of the body to be objectionable.

Others object to cremation on environmental principles, noting that the cremation of a body contributes to air pollution, releases carbon dioxide into the atmosphere, and utilizes significant amounts of energy. One estimate is that the cremation of a single body releases more than 530 pounds of carbon dioxide into the atmosphere and requires approximately the same amount of energy as two automobile tanks of gasoline. Even with some newer cremation techniques in use in India, a single open-air cremation still consumes at least 220 pounds of wood, a reduction from more traditional methods which could consume up to 1,100 pounds (Little, 2016, 2019).

When there is not a cultural or religious motivation for a particular means of disposing of the body, preferences among consumers appear to be changing. In a recent survey of 1,500 Americans, 29% indicated they planned a traditional burial and 37% indicated they would opt for cremation. Both of these numbers were lower than when the same survey was conducted three years earlier during the COVID-19 pandemic; at that time, 35% indicated they would opt for traditional burial and 44% indicated they were most interested in cremation. The remaining portion of Americans in the surveys were evenly split between the decisions for natural burial, donation to science, and lack of a plan, with the most rapid growth happening in the "natural burial" category, from 4% in 2020 to 11% in 2023 (Martin, 2023).

In many parts of the world and in European and North American history, the use of a professional funeral director is a relatively recent innovation. Prior to the mid-19th century, American families, for example, would rely on friends and extended family members to bathe, dress, and lay out the deceased while others built the coffin and dug the grave. Within a day or so of death, the funeral was held with a horse and wagon conveying the deceased from family home to graveyard, sometimes with a stop for a funeral service in the church. When the formal part of the ceremony ended, men in the community lowered the coffin into the grave that they had perhaps dug just that morning and filled it back in. Undertaking was a family and community affair (Laderman, 2005).

As more Americans moved to urban communities, space for laying out the dead at home became scarcer, and families less often had the equipment to construct their own coffins. Furniture makers undertook the role of making coffins, transporting both bodies and coffins from homes to churches and on to cemeteries. Furniture- and cabinetmakers gradually added undertaking services to their names, and many funeral homes with 19th-century roots describe on their company history website pages their beginnings as furniture stores (Laderman, 2005). At least across the United States of the mid-20th century, the movement of the dead from the family home to the funeral home was more a concession to smaller homes on crowded city streets with inadequate parking than it was any sinister move on the part of the funeral industry to hold the dead hostage, as Mitford (1963) criticized.

With the movement of funeral ceremonies and care of the dead into professional hands in Europe and North America of the mid-20th century, interest in providing families an opportunity to care for their own dead emerged, with advocates suggesting families could become their own funeral director and arrange direct cremations. Carlson (1987) surveyed laws across the United States and explained in simplified language how a family could perform these tasks, based in large measure on her own experience caring for her husband's body after his death.

Martin (2023) reported that more than 50% of American consumers would consider a do-it-yourself (DIY) funeral. Clinical experience, however, indicates that many people who hypothesize they would opt for a DIY funeral themselves may find their family unwilling or emotionally unable to carry out those tasks. Although there seem to be no reliable estimates, urban families in Europe and North America who undertake all tasks on their own without professional assistance seem to be in a very distinct minority.

A middle-ground solution began emerging in the early 1990s with accelerating interest into the early decades of the 21st century: professionally assisted simple burial. Although the level of professional assistance is varied, there seems to be growing interest in natural burial where the remains are kept at home for a day or two until a burial in a natural burial ground. When Ken West sought to return burial rites to families with the opening of the United Kingdom's first natural burial ground in Carlisle in 1993, natural burial began to experience a rebirth (Davies & Rumble, 2012). Within 30 years, more than 270 such natural burial grounds opened across the United Kingdom (Natural Death Centre, 2023).

Some funeral homes, including those certified by the Green Burial Council, agree to work with families to transport and shelter remains, provide a gathering space for services, and offer a selection of biodegradable caskets. In most cases, families can be as involved as desired in the preparations and carrying out of the funeral.

"Natural burial" is defined in various ways, but in general, it implies that the body is cared for with a minimum amount of professional care that is typically included in a funeral home's basic services. For example, natural burial advocates eschew embalming with formaldehyde and other toxic chemicals, preferring to temporarily retard decomposition with the use of ice packs around the remains.

Bedino (2009) wrote about the procedures of ecobalming, providing preservation using 21st-century injection embalming techniques but utilizing fluids that are environmentally friendly. The effect of this process, he wrote, is that temporary retarding of decomposition becomes evident immediately, permitting the remains to be held for three to five days or even longer if the body is refrigerated after treatment. Ecobalming is intended to temporarily delay the process of the body returning to its natural elements and provides an alternative to the odors and discoloration typical of bodies that have not been embalmed.

Natural burial almost always includes burial in a simple fabric shroud or wicker basket without rigid caskets, vaults, and grave liners so that the body more easily disintegrates in the soil. Some of these natural burial sites do not utilize grave markers, instead relying on GPS coordinates to locate graves. Other sites are more flexible, perhaps permitting markers as long as they are made from natural stone and not mounted in concrete (Yang, 2023).

There are a multitude of national natural burial associations, any of which can be found through an internet search. New Zealand's Natural Burials and the United States' Green Burial Council each lists certified funeral providers and natural cemeteries across their respective countries. Australia's Natural Death Advocacy Network, Canada's Natural Burial Association of Ontario, and the United Kingdom's Natural Death Centre all provide resources and links to natural burial grounds in their respective jurisdictions. Other countries have growing natural burial movements including the Netherlands and France (Tschebann, 2022).

The use of cadavers in medical research and teaching is as old as medical education itself, likely dating to the third or fourth century B.C.E. However, the choice of individuals to donate their body to science gained new life with the codification of the Uniform Anatomical Gift Act of 1968, standardizing procedures for whole-body donation (Sadler et al., 1968). Typically referred to as willed body programs, many medical schools accept donations based on the school's needs for research and dissection in anatomy labs. In recent years, for-profit companies have also arisen that accept bodies for scientific research, though some of these organizations have come under increasing scrutiny because of their tendency to dissect bodies and send parts to different research institutions. Donors and their families will want to research options in the geographical region where death is expected since most medical school willed body programs seem to provide only local transportation from the place of death. Codes of ethics and other guidelines are emerging in this rapidly changing arena (American Association for Anatomy, 2023).

As environmental concerns continued to grow related to cremation and its use of resources, innovators devised a process of dissolving the body in liquid, which can then be disposed of through the wastewater discharge system into municipal sewers. Alkaline hydrolysis, sometimes referred to as "water cremation," utilizes a combination of water and alkaline chemicals, which are placed in a sealed tank along with the body. Typically, the chamber is heated and the contents are agitated to accelerate the decomposition process. The resulting bone fragments are removed and dried before being pulverized to place in an urn and the remaining effluent is discharged with wastewater (Cremation Association of North America, 2023b).

The process is applauded by its advocates for accomplishing the same end results as cremation except that the body's water and fat are converted into wastewater instead of discharged into the atmosphere through flame-based crematory smoke. In 2010, the Cremation Association of North America (2023b) amended its definition of cremation to include both flame-based cremation and water-based cremation (alkaline hydrolysis) to allow its policies to more nearly reflect state and provincial laws already in effect.

Natural organic reduction, or human composting, borrows from a long-used technology to compost dead livestock. Human composting utilizes a tightly controlled process to reduce the body to its basic organic elements. The body is first placed in a vat of wood chips, alfalfa, and straw. Then, through the introduction of additional heat and oxygen, microbes do their natural work of decomposing the soft tissues in a period of a month or two. Typically, the bones are extracted during the process, ground into smaller particles, and returned to the developing compost. Advocates say that at the end of the process, also known as terramation, about one cubic yard of composted soil is delivered to the bereaved family when the process is complete (Helmore, 2023; Yang, 2023).

Judaism and Islam, along with many traditional Christian groups, have long-encouraged simple, natural burials. Their belief systems encourage the body to be returned to the earth from which it came, an application of what these groups see in their scriptures (Genesis 3:19; Ecclesiastes 3:20). However, whereas natural burial of the entire human body in a specific, permanent place is encouraged by most religious groups, some resist human composting because of their beliefs about the sanctity of the body.

The U.S. Conference of Catholic Bishops (2023), for example, expressed its opinion that the Roman Catholic Church's doctrine about the need for respecting the "bodily remains of the deceased in a way that gives visible witness to our faith and hope in the resurrection of the body. Unfortunately . . . alkaline hydrolysis and human composting fail to meet this criterion" (p. 4). The bishops went on to explain that the reason for their opposition to these newly emerging technologies was the same as the Church's opposition to the scattering of cremated remains: that the Church expects the remains to be placed together in a sacred place such as a cemetery or church to await the final resurrection.

Memorial Merchandise

A plethora of products have been developed seemingly as means to help bereaved individuals and families navigate the grief process in a more meaningful way (Dickinson, 2012). Interestingly, many of these items were developed by bereaved family members as a means to invest their own creativity into the memorial ceremonies to make them more personally meaningful. The products that have been developed in recent years are undoubtedly available because easy access to technology has made them easier to create quickly and often at reasonably low cost.

Before the 1990s, families making funeral arrangements virtually anywhere in the world would have chosen from a handful of standard caskets constructed of metal or wood. Depending on the funeral provider, the metal caskets would have been divided into the type and thickness of the metal with casket models available in several thicknesses of carbon steel (such as 18 gauge and 20 gauge), stainless steel, copper, and bronze. Wood caskets were most often constructed of pine, poplar, pecan, or oak with some fine caskets available in maple, cherry, and mahogany.

Traditionally, caskets made from less expensive species of wood such as pine and poplar as well as from 20 gauge carbon steel were available at a much lower price than the other models described. Most funeral providers have traditionally also offered at least a few caskets that were made with cloth-covered pressed wood or fiberboard that would have been available at a much lower price than either the least expensive steel or wood varieties in an attempt to provide something for every family's ability to pay (Private Label Caskets, 2023). Although the research for this book did not specifically address casket options, interviews with funeral directors often included visits to the funeral home's selection room (sometimes called the memorial products room or the memorial gallery) and discussions of what families are choosing in the second decade of the 21st century.

According to funeral director interviewees who had been in the profession for several decades, the consensus has been that the early 1990s was when the shift began to occur as families demanded a higher level of personal customization in the caskets chosen. In those early years of customization, if a family wanted to have a casket customized, the options would include such things as having a personalized insert developed that could be placed inside the open lid of the casket. Several older funeral directors talked of having a local embroiderer who might stitch a name or personal message on the casket throw, the piece of interior-matching fabric that made a half-open casket (called a half couch) appear more "finished."

Eventually, casket manufacturers began to develop interchangeable casket head panels with embroidered art or wording such as a rose with the words "Beloved Mom." Several leading casket manufacturers developed interchangeable corner emblems that represented a near-infinite number of faith perspectives, hobbies, and career pursuits with three-dimensional emblems such as praying hands, golf clubs, fishing motifs, and even the mortar and pestle of a pharmacist (Batesville Casket Company, 2022; Matthews Aurora Funeral Solutions, 2023).

Several funeral director respondents indicated that they regularly have families choose some level of customization of the casket ranging from a simple laser engraving of a name on a casket to fully customized caskets and urns. Technology in the first decades of the 21st century has made it possible for families to choose highly customized caskets with "wrap designs" in a number of motifs from outdoors to gardening to service branches such as Marine Corps or firefighter themes. One of the manufacturers of these highly artistic approaches to personalizing caskets displays an online photo gallery featuring caskets customized on vinyl media printed with such images as sports team logos, university themes, Spiderman and other comic characters, butterflies, and dozens of other designs. Their website declares that their "casket wraps" allow families to "visually express the life they lived" (https://wewrapcaskets.com/).

Caskets have apparently not been the only burial products families have expected to customize with personalized photographs and artwork. Since many cemeteries require a reinforced rigid burial vault around the casket to ensure the grave does not eventually collapse, one of North America's leading burial vault manufacturers, Wilbert Funeral Solutions, has responded with a customized line of burial vault lids that are personalized with a collage of photos from the deceased person's life. The company notes in its promotional website about the product that this level of customization helps to "celebrate spirituality, family, passion, life with a treasured tribute" (Wilbert Funeral Solutions, 2023, n.p.).

In the same way that there is a dizzying array of casket choices and customizations available, so it is also true with cremation urns. Urn manufacturer catalogs and websites offer thousands of choices. Because they are smaller than burial caskets, some funeral consumers find it much easier to consider purchasing an urn online than they would a larger, more-difficult-to-ship item such as a burial casket. Cremation urns are manufactured using a diversity of materials including resins, metal alloys, hardwoods, sheet bronze, stained glass, and cloisonne overlaying steel (North American Urns and Memorials, 2023).

Like those for every other consumer product, urn websites and brochures tout the benefits of their products. The website of one Australian manufacturer, for example, painstakingly explains the virtues of the various species of wood from which the company's urns are constructed, explaining the features of each one. For example, the website details the unique properties of its urns made from Australian chestnut:

> Australian Chestnut is sustainably harvested from several different Eucalypt species. This timber is prized for its unique markings caused by bushfires, environmental conditions and insects. We source wood that showcases these markings, giving your urn a visible history of the individual tree.
>
> (Urns of Distinction, 2023, n.p.)

Although it first became popular in the 19th century, memorial jewelry has risen in popularity in recent years. Bereavement professionals recognize that the goal of grief is less about a Freudian "disconnection" from the dead so that one can "move on with life" and more about a sense of "continuing bond" with the deceased in some spiritual and emotional sense (Klass, 2006; Klass et al., 1996). Maintaining some physical connection to the deceased might be the psychological reality behind placing flowers on a grave in a cemetery visit or maintaining a roadside memorial where a loved one died. The same impulse toward physical proximity might account for the resurgence in recent years of memorial jewelry.

Queen Victoria (1819–1901) famously sent snippets of Prince Albert's hair to Garrard, the royal jeweler, after her husband's death so it could be made into memorial jewelry. Garrard made at least eight such pieces of jewelry for the queen including a gold-and-onyx hairpin. The royal couple's eight-year-old son was required to wear a locket containing "beloved Papa's hair" (Lutz, 2011, p. 132). However, Victoria did not invent the custom but rather seemed to have adapted it from the use of mourning jewelry among the aristocracy in 18th-century England and France (Tsoumas, 2023).

In similar ways, some contemporary memorial products seem to have less to do with the ceremonies surrounding death than maintaining this physical proximity with the deceased. In the opening decades of the 21st century, "cremation jewelry" seems to help address this need. One bereaved mother explained that she kept most of her son's cremated remains in an urn at home but that she also wore a cremation pendant shaped like a heart around her neck. Her explanation of the simple necklace was straightforward: "I always want to feel I have him close to my heart."

"Keepsake urns," which allow family members to divide up the deceased's cremated remains among several family members, may play a similar role in the bereavement experience. A funeral director informant explained how one family purchased seven of these miniature urns so that each of the deceased's six children and his wife could each have a small portion of cremated remains. The family gathered at a lake and scattered the remains that did not fit into the seven keepsake urns at "John's favorite fishing spot."

In addition to pendants and lockets designed to contain a small portion of the cremated remains, memorial jewelry includes items such as pendants with the deceased person's fingerprint engraved on a piece of 14k gold or sterling silver jewelry. One such pendant includes an optional birthstone so that the deceased's birth month and fingerprint are melded into a single keepsake. Although interviews indicate these "fingerprint keepsakes" have grown significantly, there can be concerns about legal issues if a funeral provider is perceived to be "invading privacy" (Logan, 2023, p. 98).

Placing cremated remains in an urn or cremation jewelry are two options for cremated remains, but there is no shortage of creativity families display in creating new ways to permanently memorialize their loved ones. Cremated remains can be mixed with color pigments for the ink to create memorial tattoos, pressed into synthetic gemstones, blended with the vinyl used to produce phonograph records, and mixed with clay to be cast into pottery (Little, 2016). Although some of these options potentially utilize the entire eight pounds or so of cremated remains, options such as the tattoo ink use a tiny portion, so families must decide what to do with the remainder.

One funeral director described the interaction with a family who wanted to memorialize their young adult son who had always said he wanted his cremated remains launched in fireworks shells in a colorful show at the water's edge. At the time (the early 1990s), the funeral director had never heard of such a plan, but there was time as the young man was dying from a debilitating illness. By the time of his death, a vendor had been secured who packed the cremated remains in enough fireworks shells for a grand 20-minute display. Family watched from a nearby boat while friends gathered on the beach. A few days later at the young man's memorial service, still photos from the fireworks bursts were shown in the tribute slide show that concluded the memorial service.

Bereaved families also seek out a diversity of other memorial products from a funeral home, a cremation center, or an online vendor. Most funeral homes visited displayed a dozen or more options for memorial guest books from which a bereaved family could choose, but an internet search for "funeral guest books" revealed hundreds of options from which buyers could select, including some that could be shipped overnight with the deceased's name and photo custom printed on the cover.

Lingering Questions about Funeral Effectiveness

The vast array of services and memorial merchandise available whereby a newly bereaved individual and family may commemorate the life and death of a loved one, paired with questions raised in Chapter 5 about the economic costs of arranging services leads to an important question: Is there any enduring value to funeral services and merchandise in the long-term bereavement outcomes of bereaved family members and community? Most studies point to a positive effect on bereavement outcomes when families have participated in personally meaningful memorial ceremonies in which they played the role they desired and in which they derived satisfaction that the service was in line with their own preferences (Castle & Phillips, 2003; Fristad et al., 2001; Gamino et al., 2000; Hoy, 2013; Wijngaards-de Meij et al., 2008).

Two recent studies have raised questions about the efficacy of memorial ceremonies, both of which specifically considered cremation ceremonies. Birrell and colleagues (2020) conducted a longitudinal study to examine the responses of 263 bereaved individuals across the United Kingdom to ascertain the correlations between the cremation arrangements and services in which the respondents participated and their bereavement outcomes at two distinct time periods. The researchers acknowledged earlier theoretical perspectives and research that supported the connection between funeral arrangements chosen and bereavement outcomes, several of which the study authors acknowledged were summarized in Hoy (2013). In light of these earlier perspectives on funeral options, these researchers sought to understand how cremation services, and especially the recent growth of so-called direct cremation, in the United Kingdom might affect bereavement outcomes. They utilized a series of questions to determine the components of the cremation chosen and the Inventory of Complicated Grief–Revised to evaluate the levels of bereavement symptomatology experienced by respondents.

In the first survey, respondents were from two to five months post-loss, and at the second survey, respondents were between 14 and 17 months post-loss. With an 11.4% attrition rate between T^1 and T^2, researchers found that there were "no particularly outstanding, notable or impactful relationships" between the cremation services chosen and the levels of grief during their survey period (Birrell et al., 2020, p. 384).

Based on the results of correlating the types of services in which individuals participated and their bereavement experiences over time, the researchers concluded that "it does not matter to grief whether a more minimalistic or elaborate funeral ceremony was observed." Because these results seem contrary to both received wisdom and earlier studies, the authors advised caution when interpreting the data or suggesting causality. The authors noted, for example, that approximately 5% of funeral arrangements in the United Kingdom involve what is commonly called direct cremation (Birrell et al., 2020, p. 372). Of the 233 respondents, 17 (7%) indicated they had arranged such a service. Although the percentage of respondents in the study arranging a direct cremation closely parallels the general memorial-arranging population, this seems to be a relatively small number on which to base a contrary theoretical position.

Although they acknowledged few individuals in their study with experiences of problematic grief, Mitima-Verloop et al. (2021) similarly found no significant association between the use of funeral rituals and long-term bereavement outcomes. In their sample, 552 Dutch individuals completed questionnaires at six months post-loss, and 289 completed questionnaires at three years post-loss. Even though there was no statistical correlation between services chosen and grief scores, participants expressed a high level of endorsement of the idea that the funeral ceremonies helped the bereaved in processing their loss (75.9% at six months; 70.2% at three years) (p. 739). In concert with earlier research (Possick et al., 2007), the researchers suggested that public rituals seem to be more important in cases of sudden and unexpected death where meaning making is defined in collective terms rather than rituals being simply a means to personal "emotional catharsis" (Mitima-Verloop et al., 2021, p. 742).

Mitima-Verloop and colleagues (2021) acknowledged limitations to their study including how the sample was identified. As reported, however, the research did not include a nuanced study of types of collective memorial rituals other than inquiring of whether the respondent participated in a memorial ceremony, and if so, what level of satisfaction that ceremony held for the bereaved individual. These measures do not provide a proxy for the details of the collective rituals arranged and their relative helpfulness or lack of helpfulness in the long-term bereavement adjustment. Therefore, it is difficult to generalize these results.

Clinical Implications

Although there is wide consensus among bereavement clinicians and researchers about the likely usefulness of memorial rituals in helping bereaved individuals navigate the grief process, one cannot definitively conclude on the basis of empirical evidence that funerals are vital or that a certain kind of funeral is best. Both Birrell and colleagues (2020) and Mitima-Verloop and colleagues (2021) underscored the clinical importance of inquiring about how satisfied the bereaved individual was with the memorial options selected and how the bereaved individual perceives the helpfulness of the rituals. This seems to be the most important area in which to initiate conversation about the rituals chosen and how the bereaved individual wishes those ceremonies would have been different.

The wide range of memorial service options and products, including many that are widely available to individuals online, may provide clinicians with ample suggestions for creating personally meaningful ceremonies and tribute keepsakes, even long after the death and the formal collective memorial rituals have been held. Clinicians can suggest and even cocreate memorial items with bereaved individuals as part of the therapeutic process and the wide variety of these items would likely expand the usefulness of therapeutic rituals in grief counseling suggested in earlier studies and theoretical perspectives (Castle & Philips, 2003; Neimeyer, 2012, 2015; Rando, 1985, Reeves, 2011; Sas & Coman, 2016; Worden, 2018).

Reflection and Discussion

- Which method of body disposition is of greatest interest to you? How did you make that choice? How do you think your own family and community would applaud or oppose your decision?
- What memorialization merchandise options do you find most creative? What would you add to the list if you were a "memorial inventor"?
- How would you help a family negotiate compromise, achieve consensus, and reach agreement when different members of the family advocate or oppose particular methods of body disposition or memorialization?

References

American Association for Anatomy. (2023). Body donation policy. https://www.anatomy.org.

Arnold, D. (2016). Burning issues: Cremation and incineration in modern India. *Naturwissenschaften, Technik und Medizin*, 24(4), 393–419. https://doi.org/10.1007/s00048-017-0158-7.

Australian Museum. (2018). Burial—Coffins and caskets. https://australian.museum/.

Batesville Casket Company. (2022). Remember every story. https://cdn.batesville.com/uploads/2022/05/Family-Choices-Personalization-Brochure-US-March-2022.pdf.

Bedino, J.H. (2009). Ecobalming with *Enigma*: The champion guide to green embalming practices and postmortem preparation of bodies for natural/green burial and ecocremation/disposition. *Champion Expanding Encyclopedia of Mortuary Practices*, 658, 2717–2724. https://thechampioncompany.com/content/pdfs/encyclo658.pdf.

Birrell, J., Schut, H., Stroebe, M., Anadria, D., Newsom, C., Woodthorpe, K., Rumble, H., Corden, A., & Smith, Y. (2020). Cremation and grief: Are ways of commemorating the dead related to adjustment over time? *Omega: Journal of Death & Dying*, 81(3), 370–392. https://doi.org/10.1177/0030222820919253.

Bonn-Muller, E. (2009). Entombed in style. *Archaeology*, 62(3), 40–43.

Brooten, D., Youngblut, J.M., Charles, D., Roche, R., Hidalgo, I., & Malkawi, F. (2016). Death rituals reported by white, Black, and Hispanic parents following the ICU death of an infant or child. *Journal of Pediatric Nursing*, 31(2), 132–140. https://doi.org/10.1016/j.pedn.2015.10.017.

Carlson, L. (1987). *Caring for your own dead*. Upper Access Publishers.

Castle J., & Phillips, W.L. (2003). Grief rituals: Aspects that facilitate adjustment to bereavement. *Journal of Loss & Trauma*, 8, 41–71. https://www.doi.org/10.1080/15325020305876.

CE Noticias Financieras. (2020, October 31). During the pandemic cremations increase in Mexico [*Durante la pandemia aumentan las cremaciones en México*]. *ProQuest Wire Services*. https://www.proquest.com.

CEIC Data. (2023). China funeral service: Cremation rate. https://www.ceicdata.com/en/china/funeral-service-overview/cn-funeral-service-cremation-rate.

Cremation Association of North America. (2023a). Alkaline hydrolysis. https://www.cremationassociation.org/page/alkalinehydrolysis.

Cremation Association of North America. (2023b). Cremation process. https://www.cremationassociation.org/page/CremationProcess/.

Curry, A. (2020, November 23). "Death has become a big business." Elaborate coffins illuminate the hidden history of ancient Egypt. *Science*. https://www.science.org.

Davies, D.J., & Rumble, H. (2012). *Natural burial: Traditional-secular spiritualities and funeral innovation*. Continuum.

Dickinson, G.E. (2012). Diversity in death: Body disposition and memorialization. *Illness, Crisis & Loss*, 20, 141–158. https://www.doi.org/10.2190/IL.20.2.d.

Dlábiková, I., Peřinková, M., & Kovář, J. (2022). Brief history of crematoria and mourning halls. Modern cremation history. *Architectus, 2(70)*. https://doi.org/10.37190/arc220203.

Fristad, M.A., Cerel, J., Goldman, M., Weller, E.B., & Weller, R.A. (2001). The role of ritual in children's bereavement. *Omega: Journal of Death and Dying*, 42(4), 321–339. https://doi.org/10.2190/MC87-GQMC-VCDV-UL3U.

Gamino, L.A., Easterling, L.W., Stirman, L.S., & Sewell, K.W. (2000). Grief adjustment as influenced by funeral participation and occurrence of adverse funeral events. *Omega: Journal of Death and Dying*, 41, 79–92. https://www.doi.org/10.2190/QMV2-3NT5-BKD5-6AAV.

Hager, A. (2023, March 23). Funeral directors in 15 states can now offer the eco-friendlier "water cremation." *NPR All Things Considered*. https://npr.org/.

Helmore, E. (2023, January 1). New York governor legalizes human composting after death. *The Guardian*. https://www.theguardian.com.

Hoy, W.G. (2013). *Do funerals matter? The purposes and practices of death rituals in global perspective*. Routledge.

Kelly, S. (2015). *Greening death: Reclaiming burial practices and restoring our tie to the earth*. Rowman & Littlefield.

Klass, D. (2006). Continuing conversation about continuing bonds. *Death Studies*, 30(9), 843–858. https://doi.org/10.1080/07481180600886959.

Klass, D., Silverman, P.R., & Nickman, S.L. (Eds.). (1996). *Continuing bonds: New understandings of grief*. Taylor & Francis/Routledge.

Laderman, G. (2005). *Rest in peace: A cultural history of death and the funeral home in twentieth-century America*. Oxford University Press. https://doi.org/10.1093/acprof:oso/9780195183559.001.0001.

Little, B. (2016, May 6). Creative things to do with a dead body. *National Geographic*. https://www.nationalgeographic.com.

Little, B. (2019, November 5). The environmental toll of cremating the dead. *National Geographic*. https://www.nationalgeographic.com.

Liu, G. (2022, April 2). Why Chinese burn paper on tomb-sweeping day. *Beijinger*. https://www.thebeijinger.com/.

Logan, B. (2023). Fingerprint keepsake legality: What you need to know. *American Funeral Director*, 146(9), 96–98.

Lutz, D. (2011). The dead still among us: Victorian secular relics, hair jewelry, and death culture. *Victorian Literature and Culture*, 39(1), 127–142. https://doi.org/10.1017/S1060150310000306 4.

Martin, A. (2023, July 6). 2023 survey results: Inflation's impact on American funeral decisions. *ChoiceMutual Insurance Company*. https://choicemutual.com/blog/funeral-preferences/.

Matthews Aurora Funeral Solutions. (2023). Burial caskets: Personalization. https://matthewsaurora.com/products/burial-products/personalization/.

Mitford, J. (1963). *The American way of death*. Simon & Schuster.

Mitima-Verloop, H.B., Mooren, T.T.M., & Boelen, P.A. (2021). Facilitating grief: An exploration of the function of funerals and rituals in relation to grief reactions. *Death Studies*, 45(9), 735–745. https://doi.org/10.1080/07481187.2019.1686090.

Mylonas, G.E. (1948). Homeric and Mycenaean burial customs. *American Journal of Archaeology*, 52(1), 56–81. https://doi.org/10.2307/500553.

Natural Death Centre. (2023). Association of Natural Burial Grounds: An introduction. www.naturaldeath.org.uk.

Neimeyer, R.A. (Ed.). (2012). *Techniques of grief therapy: Creative practices for counseling the bereaved*. Routledge.

Neimeyer, R.A. (Ed.). (2015). *Techniques of grief therapy: Assessment and intervention*. Routledge.

North American Urns and Memorials. (2023). Cremation urns. https://northamericanurns.com/collections.

Possick, C., Buchbinder, E., Etzion, L., Yehoshua-Halevi, A., Fishbein, S., & Nissim-Frankel, M. (2007). Reconstructing the loss: Hantzacha commemoration following the death of a spouse in a terror attack. *Journal of Loss & Trauma*, 12(2), 111–126. https://doi.org/10.1080/15325020600945947.

Private Label Caskets. (2023). Casket collection. https://privatelabelcaskets.com/pages/casket-collections.

Prothero, S. (2001). *Purified by fire: A history of cremation in America*. University of California Press. https://doi.org/10.1525/j.ctt1pnnhg.

Ramos-de Viesca, M., Avila, M.E., Chiapas, M.G., de los Angeles González, M., & Pérez, L. (2002). Cremation. A public health chapter in Mexico [*La cremación. Un capítulo en la salud pública de México*]. *Gaceta Médica de México*, 138(6), 581–586. https://www.medigraphic.com/cgi-bin/new/resumen.cgi?IDARTICULO=7576.

Rando, T.A. (1985). Creating therapeutic rituals in the psychotherapy of the bereaved. *Psychotherapy: Theory, Research, Practice, Training*, 22, 236–240. https://doi.org/10.1037/h0085500.

Reeves, N.C. (2011). Death acceptance through ritual. *Death Studies*, 35(5), 408–419. https://doi.org/10.1080/07481187.2011.552056.

Rutherford, H.R. (2001). *Honoring the dead: Catholics and cremation today*. Liturgical Press.

Sadler, A.M., Sadler, B.L., & Stason, E.B. (1968). The Uniform Anatomical Gift Act: A model for reform. *Journal of the American Medical Association*, 206(11), 2501–2506. https://doi.org/10.1001/jama.1968.03150110049007.

Sas, C., & Coman, A. (2016). Designing personal grief rituals: An analysis of symbolic objects and actions. *Death Studies*, 40(9), 558–569. https://doi.org/10.1080/07481187.2016.1188868.

Thompson, H. (1891). *Modern cremation: Its history and practice with information relating to the recently improved arrangements made by the Cremation Society of England*. Kegan Paul, Trench, Trubner.

Tschebann, S. (2022). Cemetery enchanted, Encore: Natural burial in France and beyond. In E. Weiss-Krejci, S. Becker, & P. Schwyzer (Eds.), *Interdisciplinary explorations of postmortem interaction* (pp. 249–268). Springer. https://doi.org/10.1007/978-3-031-03956-0_11.

Tsoumas, J. (2023). Mourning jewelry in late Georgian and Victorian Britain: A world of fantasy and tears. *Convergências*, 15(30), 121–134. https://doi.org/10.53681/c1514225187514391s.30.150.

Urns of Distinction. (2023). Timbers used in cremation urns. https://urnsofdistinction.com.au/timbers/.

U.S. Conference of Catholic Bishops, Committee on Doctrine. (2023, March 20). On the proper disposition of bodily remains. https://www.usccb.org/resources/On%20Proper%20Disposition%202023-03-20.pdf.

Wijngaards-de Meij, L., Stroebe, M.S., Stroebe, W., Schut, H.A.W., Bout, J., Van der Heijden, P.G., & Dijkstra, I.C. (2008). The impact of circumstances surrounding the death of a child on parents' grief. *Death Studies*, 32, 237–252. doi:10.1080/07481180701881263.

Wilbert Funeral Solutions. (2023). Wilbert legacy custom prints. https://www.wilbert.com.

Worden, J.W. (2018). *Grief counseling and grief therapy: A handbook for the mental health practitioner* (5th ed.). Springer.

Yang, A. (2023, February 29). Rest in . . . compost? These "green funerals" offer an eco-friendly afterlife. *National Geographic*. https://www.nationalgeographic.com.

Epilogue

Twice in my own family, we experienced deaths in the same family branch in a period of only 13 months. Daniel Ray Hoy (1981–2020), my brother's eldest son, was 38 years old when he died suddenly—and not—at the end of more than three decades of living with Duchenne muscular dystrophy. His obituary declared the young man's indomitable spirit: "Though he was wheelchair-bound after age 8, he never let his disability stop him; the passion with which he lived life was captured in the name he gave his blog, 'Rolling with the Punches'" (Legacy.com, 2020).

Daniel's death in the teeth of the global COVID-19 pandemic on August 14, 2020 caused some consternation to his parents as they thought about his funeral. For a decade, Don, Daniel's dad and my brother, had pastored the Southside Baptist Church in Denham Springs, Louisiana. Because the town lay just across the Amite River from the sprawling urban area of Baton Rouge, this placed Denham Springs in a different parish (county) with less restrictive gathering restrictions than in the much larger urban parish to the east. Choosing a funeral home in Denham Springs rather than Baton Rouge would prove fortuitous for how Daniel's funeral services could unfold. Guests would be expected to remain masked indoors, and the rows of chairs in the funeral chapel were set several feet apart, but otherwise, there was no limit on the number of family and friends who could participate in Daniel's services. In the neighboring community, the family would have been limited to only ten guests, which would not even have included the entire extended family.

When Don called to tell me of Daniel's death, I left almost immediately to drive the eight hours from my home in Texas to Daniel's family's home. Over the next week, I walked with my brother's family through the experiences of loss, helped them arrange the details of the funeral, and stood with them around Daniel's casket as they viewed his body for the first time since his death. Although significantly atrophied by the ravages of the disease that ended Daniel's life, his legs were covered by the same LSU Tigers blanket I had seen dozens of times in his lap as he sat in his powered wheelchair. It

DOI: 10.4324/9781003353010-11

was a fitting remembrance for a man who loved LSU athletics—in both the good years and the lean ones.

During the evening's visitation, I worked the crowd, greeting the more than 80 people in line at any one time across the corridor of the funeral home waiting to pay their respects and speak to Don and Susan. I heard story after story of the indomitable spirit of this young man and the impact he had on so many patients and families, at home and around the world. One man who drove several hours to join our family had been in Daniel's school class the day he walked for the last time. We had already heard about the Facebook post from the mother of a Duchenne patient in the United Kingdom for whom Daniel had demonstrated such concern and compassion after her own son died.

Daniel's life was characterized by his strong faith, and that was clear in the perspective his family penned for the newspaper obituary. In that obituary, his family wrote,

> On Friday morning, Jesus pointed to the wheelchair sitting by his bed and said, "Hey Daniel. You won't be needing this anymore. Enough is enough. Come on home with Me." Though our hearts are broken, they are also overwhelmed with joy that he is running on the streets of gold with Jesus and breathing on his own, free from the constraints of a body that continued to fail him. "We grieve . . . but not as others who have no hope" (1 Thessalonians 4:13).
>
> (Legacy.com, 2020)

The funeral home chapel was packed full of people as the hour approached for Daniel's service to begin that Friday morning. Strains of contemporary Christian music, the genre Daniel loved best, filled the room as photos from his life flashed on the screen above the casket. Daniel's dad—and my brother—Don, addressed the crowd to welcome the mourners and express the gratitude of his family. Then he took his seat next to Susan, and then I stepped to the microphone to read from the scriptures so essential to our family's faith.

The scripture I read seemed appropriate for the occasion of the funeral of a man who had not walked on his own legs since he was eight years old, though in our family's confident faith, now "ran free":

> Have you not known? Have you not heard? The Lord is the everlasting God, the Creator of the ends of the earth. He does not faint or grow weary; his understanding is unsearchable. . . . Even youths shall faint and be weary, and young men shall fall exhausted; but they who wait for the Lord shall renew their strength; they shall mount up

> with wings like eagles; they shall run and not be weary, they shall walk and not faint.
>
> (Isaiah 40:28–31, ESV)

Then three pastors in turn, each of them who had been friends of Don's and Susan's in their seminary days nearly four decades earlier, led the remainder of the funeral service to minister to the gathered mourners. After all of the friends in attendance had been ushered out to their cars, the family spent a few minutes together around Daniel's casket and each said their tearful goodbyes to his physical remains.

Following the funeral service, family and friends were escorted by police officers from multiple jurisdictions in procession to the cemetery ten miles away where Daniel was buried in the last grave plot his grandparents—our parents—had purchased for their own use in 1956. He was buried in a plot adjoining the grandparents he loved, near his great-grandparents whom he had never met since the last of them died 15 years before Daniel's birth. In his burial site, there was a "continuity with the generations."

The experience of grief was hard. There were ups and downs over the following year, but for everyone involved, the conclusion was unanimous that their bereavement was immeasurably easier because there had been an opportunity to say goodbye through a funeral. Although no one felt particularly guilty about the choices, we were deeply mindful that most families did not enjoy the luxury of creating a ceremony in the midst of the pandemic that our family created. Other than seats being more spaced apart in the funeral chapel and the use of masks indoors, the funeral was largely unrestricted.

Little could any of us have known the day we laid my nephew to rest that our family would face the rigors of a funeral ceremony again not quite 13 months later when his dad died from a COVID-19 infection. Don spent the last 30 days of his life in the hospital with the final two weeks in the intensive care unit on a ventilator. Now the pandemic touched our family's life in a way none of us had been impacted until that moment.

Although Don's early prognosis for recovery seemed good, in retrospect our family has acknowledged that he was emotionally worn-out by grieving his son's death, coupled by the physical depletion of having been a full-time family caregiver to Daniel for many years in addition to his congregational duties. The emotional and physical exhaustion along with the virulent infection simply proved too much for his 63-year-old body to withstand. In the wee hours of September 9, 2021, our family's belief is that Don went directly into the presence of his Lord and joined his son. Don's daughter, Stephanie, pictured it as Daniel running to greet his dad "on the other shore."

By the early fall of 2021, pandemic restrictions had eased considerably in southern Louisiana, but the region reeled from two hurricanes that made landfall back to back. Coupled with an upsurge in deaths and a backlog in the funeral home due to the burial delays brought about from the storms, it would be nine days from Don's death until we could hold his funeral. Nevertheless, we were grateful that in south Louisiana, we were able to hold a "normal funeral" at all since so much of the United States and the world were still under significant restrictions.

The Friday evening visitation would be held in the sanctuary of the congregation Don served, even though we knew intuitively the seating capacity of the little church would be far too small for the expected attendance at the Saturday morning funeral service. A couple of hundred people came by on Friday evening to pay their respects and to offer support to Susan and her family. Like with most "traditional" funeral visitations, this one offered people an opportunity to express their sadness and to tell stories of how Don had cared for them.

Through the evening, I heard multiple tales of how Don had given so much to so many people. The stories included the man who told of how Don waited with him at the hospital when his wife was undergoing surgery, and they included the woman who recounted how Don had been with them in the wee hours of the night when her own father had died. Again and again, our family heard the many ways our husband, father, and brother had been there for others, making an indelible imprint on the lives of so many. As the pastor of small, mostly rural congregations for nearly four decades, Don's name had never really been in the lights, but it was clear that his life had been a light for hundreds of people.

That impact became especially evident on Saturday morning as more than 375 people gathered in the nearby First Baptist Church of Denham Springs. That congregation's leadership, staff, and volunteers welcomed us into their home as if we were part of their faith family. They showed us both care and hospitality and compassionately helped us navigate these difficult hours of our mourning.

About 20 uniformed officers of the Civil Air Patrol along with four cadets Don had mentored joined us for the ceremony. It seemed fitting they should be seated together in a place of honor in the front of the church, opposite our family, because they represented an important part of Don's volunteer life as he had served as their wing chaplain. The cadets stood at attention at the door of the church, straightening their backs even more and saluting as Don's casket passed through the door of the church.

Once again, the three pastor buddies from Don's seminary class led the service, just as they had walked with our family in mourning Daniel just 14 months earlier. Like at Daniel's service, I began by welcoming mourners on behalf of Susan and the rest of our family and then, from my brother's own preaching Bible, read the biblical text of Don's favorite verses of scripture:

> I beseech you therefore, brethren, by the mercies of God, that you present your bodies a living sacrifice, holy, acceptable to God, *which is* your reasonable service. And do not be conformed to this world, but be transformed by the renewing of your mind, that you may prove what *is* that good and acceptable and perfect will of God.
>
> (Romans 12:1–2, NKJV)

For so many people in attendance, the highlight of the ceremony was hearing a recording of Ray Boltz singing "Thank You." The lyrics told of the songwriter's dream of being in heaven and seeing the many people whom the subject of the song had touched with compassion and faith during life on the earth. We heard the song as if an invisible person who had preceded Don in death greeted him "on the heavenly streets," expressing gratitude for the gift of service that led to changed lives (Gaither Music TV, 2012).

When the funeral ceremony ended, we went in procession just a few miles to the cemetery where Don would be buried. A gentle rain fell adding to the sadness of the day, but the faith of this family was strong. Although we would, after the reading of scripture and more prayers, say goodbye to Don's remains there in that memorial park, our family's belief is that this parting was simply "farewell for now; see you again soon."

As this volume has sought to demonstrate, there are many ways that families and communities seek to create meaning through the rituals that accompany death. Even though some individuals think they are being "creative," many of the most creative expressions of grief through ceremonies are simply new reflections of ancient customs, traditions, and ways humans behave to light their darkest nights. Sometimes the personal faith of these families informs the ceremonies they choose; sometimes their deeply embedded ethnic or cultural heritage informs them. Most often, it is some combination of faith, culture, and practices that work in cohort with caring communities to shepherd bereaved people through the most desperately difficult days of their lives.

As this book goes to press, I am nearing the end of my fortieth year of caring for families, of walking alongside the dying and bereaved, and of teaching both my colleagues in health-care and human services as well as the next generation of these professionals how to best care for these precious souls who are mourning. Almost never in those four decades—in my clinical practice nor in my research—have I heard a bereaved person who had some kind of ceremony after a loved one died wish they had not. They may have wished to have done something differently or to have added a component to the funeral they did not think to add at the time. Sometimes they have longed to have had the courage to stand up to family pressure or cultural tradition and to have done something more personal than what they ended up doing. But what they have not told me they wished is that they would have skipped the funeral completely.

Throughout history and around the world, families and communities have marked the deaths of their loved ones with ceremonies. They have mourned together and found ways, just like my brother's family and their community did, to walk out what they cannot talk out. They have depended on the deep imagery of pictures and symbols that need no explanation to those who are present and they honor deeply held cultural beliefs, practices, and customs. In diverse ways, these families and communities take leave of the physical remains of their loved persons, sometimes burying these bodies, sometimes depositing them in the depths of the ocean, sometimes leaving them on a high hill to feed the carrion of the wild, and sometimes by consigning the body to the flames. In virtually every case, however, the early moments, hours, and days of bereavement are lit up by the ways communities help families to create meaning through ceremonies.

References

Gaither Music TV. (2012, December 6). Ray Boltz—Thank you. [Video.] https://www.youtube.com/watch?v=962RR-IEcOU.

Legacy.com. (2020, August 18). Daniel Ray Hoy obituary. https://www.legacy.com.

Index

For Product Safety Concerns and Information please contact our EU representative GPSR@taylorandfrancis.com Taylor & Francis Verlag GmbH, Kaufingerstraße 24, 80331 München, Germany

Printed and bound by CPI Group (UK) Ltd, Croydon, CR0 4YY
08/06/2025
01897002-0005